We've Got Issues

Also by Judith Warner

Hillary Clinton: The Inside Story

Newt Gingrich: Speaker to America
(BY JUDITH WARNER AND MAX BERLEY)

In and Out of Vogue
(BY GRACE MIRABELLA WITH JUDITH WARNER)

You Have the Power: How to Take Back Our Country and Restore Democracy in America
(BY HOWARD DEAN WITH JUDITH WARNER)

Perfect Madness: Motherhood in the Age of Anxiety

We've Got Issues

Children and Parents *in the* Age of Medication

JUDITH WARNER

RIVERHEAD BOOKS · *a member of Penguin Group (USA) Inc.* · *New York* · *2010*

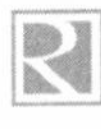

RIVERHEAD BOOKS
Published by the Penguin Group
Penguin Group (USA) Inc., 375 Hudson Street, New York, New York 10014, USA • Penguin Group (Canada), 90 Eglinton Avenue East, Suite 700, Toronto, Ontario M4P 2Y3, Canada (a division of Pearson Penguin Canada Inc.) • Penguin Books Ltd, 80 Strand, London WC2R 0RL, England • Penguin Ireland, 25 St Stephen's Green, Dublin 2, Ireland (a division of Penguin Books Ltd) • Penguin Group (Australia), 250 Camberwell Road, Camberwell, Victoria 3124, Australia (a division of Pearson Australia Group Pty Ltd) • Penguin Books India Pvt Ltd, 11 Community Centre, Panchsheel Park, New Delhi–110 017, India • Penguin Group (NZ), 67 Apollo Drive, Rosedale, North Shore 0632, New Zealand (a division of Pearson New Zealand Ltd) • Penguin Books (South Africa) (Pty) Ltd, 24 Sturdee Avenue, Rosebank, Johannesburg 2196, South Africa

Penguin Books Ltd, Registered Offices: 80 Strand, London WC2R 0RL, England

Published simultaneously in Canada

Library of Congress Cataloging-in-Publication Data

Warner, Judith.
We've got issues : children and parents in the age of medication / Judith Warner.
p. cm.
ISBN 978-1-59448-754-5
1. Child mental health–Popular works. 2. Child psychiatry–Popular works. 3. Pediatric psychopharmacology–Popular works. I. Title.
RJ499.34.W37 2010 2009040653
618.92'89–dc22

Printed in the United States of America
1 3 5 7 9 10 8 6 4 2

Book design by Claire Naylon Vaccaro

For Max, who makes everything possible

And, as always, for Julia and Emilie, with love—

Contents

Brave New World

NOUN: A world or realm of radically transformed existence, especially one in which technological progress has both positive and negative results

The American Heritage Dictionary of the English Language: Fourth Edition, 2000

Preface

As I write these pages, *Sex and the City* superstar Cynthia Nixon is starring off-Broadway in *Distracted*, a play about a mother's attempt to determine whether her son has attention-deficit/hyperactivity disorder and should be medicated. A few blocks away, the musical *Next to Normal* is putting into song a family's struggles with bipolar disorder.

In the news, a psychologist who has developed a highly regarded summer treatment program for kids with ADHD is taking on the psychiatric establishment on the safety and efficacy of stimulant medications. Federal investigators have issued a subpoena seeking detailed information about the activities of three Harvard child psychiatrists reported to have made considerable sums of money consulting for drugmakers and to have hidden much of that money from university authorities.

Meanwhile, the National Institute of Mental Health has committed $60 million in federal Recovery Act funds to autism research—the largest sum ever granted to the study of the disorder. Some mental health experts believe that in the coming decades, thanks to such research, scientists will not only be able to figure out the causes of disorders like autism, but also actually develop a possible cure.

This is a pivotal moment for mental health in America. An explosive moment. A moment pregnant with potential—for good and for ill. On the one hand, we are at the brink of never-before-seen opportunities for scientific progress. On the other hand, with these new opportunities have come terrible abuses and betrayals of the public trust. At the very least, for millions of families, there are new and difficult sorts of personal dilemmas to confront: complicated decisions, levels of confusion and pain that haven't been eased or soothed or helped or even better informed by the way we tend to talk about them in our culture at large.

Public opinion and most media treatment of this complex and confusing phenomenon have tended toward simplification. Instead of untangling the mysteries of new and confusing areas of science, teasing out what's true and untrue, good or bad about the present moment in the history of psychiatry, our culture has turned complex reality into a simple-minded morality play. In this play, the actors are defined by stereotypes, good and evil are neatly demarcated, and the truth—the gray, ambiguous truth—is deeply hidden beneath prejudice, fear, and bombast.

Nowhere is this morality play staged with greater stupidity—and cruelty—than in media depictions of how parents and doctors are caring for children with mental health issues, or, as it's generally put, "drugging" and "pathologizing" kids. In newspaper reports, TV documentaries, in the shadow world of the blogosphere, the dominant story today is one of profit-mad scientists and quick fix–seeking parents. Children, in our real and virtual watercooler chatter, are no more than misunderstood lab rats, free-spirited misfits who have to be drugged into submission because they don't conform to the demands of our competitive, hyperperformance-driven society.

When I first began this book in February 2004, I bought into that story. I was one of the many people who regarded ADHD, bipolar disorder, and the milder variants of the autistic spectrum disorders as "fashionable maladies" of questionable reality. I would, perhaps, not have been quite as blunt as Rush Limbaugh, when he described ADHD as "the perfect way to explain the inattention, incompetence, and inability of adults to control their kids," but my opinions weren't really all that far off from his views.

I am embarrassed to admit to that commonality of belief today. I cringe, thinking back on the company that I was prepared to keep, out of ignorance and a whole host of unrecognized preconceived notions about psychiatry, psychiatrists, and other parents. I really believed then that psychiatry was a sinister profession. That psychiatrists medicated kids for expediency and with a callous disregard for their unique personalities and individual life circumstances. That parents turned to psychiatry to avoid dealing with problems in their family lives that were inconvenient, or overcomplicated or, simply, embarrassing.

Writing this book changed all that.

Research, observation, scores of interviews with mental health experts, critical thinking, and, above all, the compassion I've gained from talking to dozens and dozens of the parents who stare the whole "issue" of children's mental health in the face every single day, have now made holding on to such beliefs impossible for me.

Listening to these parents, letting their voices ring out louder than the cultural noise surrounding them, a couple of simple truths have become clear.

They are: That the suffering of children with mental health issues (and their parents) is very real. That almost no parent takes the issue of psychiatric diagnosis lightly or rushes to "drug" his or her child; and that responsible child psychiatrists don't, either. And that many children's lives are essentially saved by medication, particularly when it's combined with evidence-based forms of therapy.

Saying this does not mean that I now accept absolutely everything that's done today by child psychiatrists. There is much to excoriate about the current state of psychiatric care in our country and the outsized, insufficiently regulated, sometimes criminally irresponsible role of the pharmaceutical industry.

For that matter, there is much about our current culture of childhood and the climate of contemporary family life generally that should raise alarms. These alarms have been raised many times, by many others, in the nearly endless parade of books, articles, and interviews that have been published or aired over the past few years, detailing the ways that our culture is poisoning the lives of today's kids.

I will explore all this, but, at heart, this book aims to do something different. It's an attempt to set the record straight on what life really is like for parents and children confronting mental health issues. It's an attempt to lay out what the current scientific understandings are of mental disorders. It's an attempt to get beyond hyped-up headlines and all the hand-wringing, finger-pointing, moralizing, and catastrophizing that too often dominate our discussions of children's mental health issues, and to instead start to articulate a new way to more realistically, compassionately, and productively think about and help a very vulnerable population of kids.

There's a lot of hot air circulating on the topic of children's mental health, and what the often outsized vitriol makes clear is that the passion is ideological and only tangentially about real children. Children with mental disorders have become pawns in much wider adult conflicts: about psychology versus psychiatry, about education and competition, fairness and downward mobility, about the very nature of childhood and what's generally viewed as the sorry state of modern parenting.

These are all valid and worthy topics of discussion and debate. But the way the discussion is happening now doesn't necessarily do children any good. Worrying about the state of The Child and caring for real children, after all, as all the parents interviewed here can attest, are two very different things.

• • •

Writing this book has been nothing less than an odyssey. It was a journey that went on far too long, meandered in too many wrong directions, veered at times so far off course that I thought I'd never get my feet on solid ground. But ultimately, it was the voices of the parents I met along the way that guided me toward being able to assimilate all the contradictory information that I assembled on children's mental health into a coherent and, I believe, correct story.

If you've been on a similar quest for information and understanding—and most likely, if you've known such an odyssey, it's because you yourself have a child with mental health issues—then I hope that you will find a sense of community in these pages.

If you have not, then I hope you will simply approach this book with an open mind.

There are millions of children in our country who are suffering from mental health disorders. And there is a real dividing line, a gulf of experience and understanding, that separates parents who have children with mental health issues from those who don't.

"I have found that many people think they understand depression because they have been sad," is how a mother of a boy with high-functioning autism, sensory integration issues, and obsessive behavior put it, when she wrote in to the readers' forum of "Domestic Disturbances," my online *New York Times* column, back in March, 2007. "They think they understand addiction because they have had cravings. They think they understand ADD/ADHD because they have been bored and restless. They think they understand sensory integration dysfunction because there are foods or noises they're not fond of. They think they understand obsessive-compulsive behavior because they've occasionally felt an urge to do something. The truth is that their own experiences are so far removed from the depth and magnitude of true disorders that they have no bearing on developing a better understanding of the problem."

This lack of understanding, coupled with too easy and often virulent judgments, has created a situation in which parents of children with issues feel utterly isolated. It's a situation in which, despite the fact that more help is available than ever before, parents still feel lost, families dealing with problems still are stigmatized, and our society still is not doing all that it can to give children with mental health challenges the childhood that they deserve.

If I can do something to ease that stigma, if I can make these families' experiences real for others and help pave the way toward getting them better care, then this long journey will have served a worthwhile purpose.

JUDITH WARNER
March 2009

· 1 ·

UNTITLED

on Affluent Parents and Neurotic Kids

When you embark upon a large project, it is generally a good idea to know what you are doing.

Most nonfiction books begin with a formal proposal. It lays out the book's main arguments. It provides a chapter outline. It gives a sense of how the author is going to do his or her research. It's a kind of blueprint for how to proceed.

I started this book with none of that groundwork. I didn't sell it from a proposal; I sold it from a conversation. This seemed to me to be a great triumph at the time, almost too good to be true. Which it was.

Too good to be true, I mean.

It was January of 2004. I had recently finished *Perfect Madness: Motherhood in the Age of Anxiety*, my book on the American culture of motherhood, and was in New York, having a happy lunch with my then-editor, and talking about where to pitch some magazine articles I planned to write in the year leading up to the book's publication.

One of my story ideas was on what I called the "culture of diagnosis"—the whole archipelago of therapy and tutoring and labeling and medication that I'd discovered since becoming a preschool mother in Washington,

D.C. I'd watched other moms—a lot of other moms, it seemed—dashing off with their kids to mysterious appointments in the afternoons, or having therapists in to play and swing and roll children around in tubes, and I'd found it odd and perplexing.

I didn't need to define that "culture" for my editor; she lived in it, too. We were both mothers in competitive communities, filled with high-strung, anxious parents, and kids who seemed stressed to the gills. Like most people with an opinion on the topic, contemplating a landscape of "OTs" (occupational therapists), vision therapy, brain-training software, and, especially, kids on medication, we both believed that, if so many kids around us needed such interventions, our crazy culture was making them sick. That the kids we saw making the rounds of doctors and therapies were no more than canaries in the coal mine, showing the first-line symptoms of the toxicity of our pathological age. That the helping professionals who appeared to be propagating like weeds in our communities were essentially parasites, feeding off the weakest members of our sickening world. That what lay, at base, behind all those kids' purported "issues" (as one always put it in polite conversation) was nothing more than parental—and societal—neurosis.

"Funny," my editor said, as I spelled out my idea for a magazine article that would chart the culture and business of diagnosing and treating the kids of anxious and competitive parents. "We were just saying upstairs that we were looking for someone to write a book on that topic."

My notes from the lunch contained phrases like "socially constructed illness" and "how affluent culture's anxiety disorder shows up in children."

I wrote a brief memo, and I had a book contract.

In the contract, the book was called "UNTITLED on Affluent Parents and Neurotic Kids." It was supposed to explore "fashionable children's diagnoses"—like autism, Asperger's disorder, dyslexia, attention-deficit/hyperactivity disorder, oppositional defiant disorder, anxiety disorders, and bipolar disorder—and to take aim at the "overanalyzing, the overperfecting," and "the overpathologization of America's children." Its central argument was going to be that children were, by and large, being overdiagnosed and overmedicated, and that doctors and parents and teachers and schools who colluded in labeling kids and treating them with psychotropic medication were taking the easy way out, seeking "quick fix" solutions, and turning a collective blind eye to the pathological aspects of our culture.

All systems were go.

Except that, from the very start, there was always something that blocked the book from being written.

At first, it was burnout. As I said before, I'd just finished *Perfect Madness,* and I'd sort of reached saturation point with writing and thinking about parental anxiety. I was busy with my two young daughters, and with other work.

But that was only part of the story. What really was blocking my progress was something much deeper, something that had nothing to do with *Perfect Madness* or other work. It had nothing to do with the demands of my children, or, more truthfully put, my desire to be with my children, though the "demands" of motherhood were always a convenient, and socially acceptable, excuse.

No—the problem really had to do with my book idea. Which, I started to realize when the ink on the contract was barely dry, maybe wasn't all that good.

The first sign of this came early on, again in New York, when I went to a friend's apartment to have a cup of coffee and tell her, triumphantly, about my new book.

This friend had a son who had issues. In fact, he was at that time on his way out of a mainstream private school because his issues—behavioral and emotional and learning issues—had become too much for the school to handle.

I didn't know much more about him than that at the time. I knew that he was a smart, good-looking, and athletic boy. I knew he struggled greatly with his homework and needed tutors. I knew he sometimes seemed very angry.

And I knew that his mother *did not* like the idea of my new book.

She didn't say so outright. She didn't say anything, in fact, as I went on in her living room about overdiagnosis and overmedication and the social construction of disease.

She stirred her coffee, and squared her slim shoulders.

I would later learn that her son seriously contemplated suicide at age six, had violent outbursts and paranoid episodes by age eight, and by his early teens had begun holding the family hostage to his destructive rages: breaking windows, throwing computers, punching family members, and terrifying a younger sibling, who would cower under a table for safety.

That after more than a year in residential treatment, he was able to remain at home only with the assistance of strong male "shadows," and that, when his parents tried, as they repeatedly did, to wean him off his ever-changing cocktail of antidepressants, antianxiety medications, stimulants, mood stabilizers, and antipsychotics, he'd get so much worse—paranoid, agitated, delusional—that they wondered whether he would ever be able to live on his own.

"We don't know if he will have an independent life or will be institutionalized for life," my friend would tell me, over lunch, four and a half years later, when I interviewed her for the very different book that "UNTITLED" had grown into being. "I never thought this would be my life."

In February 2004, she just fixed me with a level gaze, right about the time that I'd gotten to the part of my spiel on how the pharmaceutical industry had sold parents on drugs that didn't work.

And then she said, "*How do you know that?*"

How did I know?

Part of me bristled. How couldn't I know? The news was everywhere and had been for some time.

The headlines kept on coming: "Use of Drugs to Control Kids Worries Specialists" ("Healthy but unruly children are being given drugs for the convenience of their caretakers, not because they need them," said *The Miami Herald.*) "Pills or Patience." "The Antidepressant Dilemma." The statistics were scarier and scarier.

Prescription rates for antidepressants for kids under eighteen had more than tripled over the course of the 1990s. Stimulant use had quadrupled, and antidepressant use had also tripled.

The use of anticonvulsant medications (often prescribed to treat bipolar disorder) had nearly doubled for children and teens from 1994 to 2003.

In the same period, children's use of "atypical" antipsychotics—recently developed, powerful tranquilizing medications that had serious side effects, and had not been approved for pediatric use—had increased fivefold.

The problem wasn't just meds; globally, it seemed, kids were being grossly overpathologized, turned into psychiatric patients at the earliest possible ages.

"In New York City in the past few years, the science of early-childhood development has been pressed into service as a tool by parents and educators to correct normal variations in children's development—so that by four, or at the latest, five, they'll be prepared to compete with their kindergarten peers," said *New York* magazine, in a cover story on the city's "anxiety industry" and "culture of intervention" that ran just two months after this conversation.

The Washington Post, later that year, listed the menu of services available in Washington, D.C.'s, "Therapyland," a place, reporter Cathy Trost wrote, "familiar to any parent with a child who has problems, a theme park that woos you with the notion that the brain can be rewired and children's futures can be shaped":

> *"Some children have their own nutritionists who prescribe special supplements or diets and psychiatrists who prescribe medication for concentration, anxiety and depression. Parents hire behavioral consultants to hide in their homes and observe family dynamics, and organizational consultants, who teach kids strategies for test-taking, studying and organizing their backpacks. There are $100-an-hour consultants who will help you build a sensory-motor gym in your basement, and outfit you with special therapeutic equipment, blankets and clothes. In a search for new customers, revised versions of some therapies are marketed to 'neuro-typical' kids and adults to help enhance performance and sports skills."*

"Therapyland" was largely a place for the wealthy. Who else, after all, could afford even a portion of the $6,000 a month that, according to the *Post* piece, one Philadelphia-area family was paying to rent an apartment in the D.C. area and put their daughter through fifteen hours a week of intensive therapies and activities that included occupational therapy, language and reading therapy, vision training, Interactive Metronome therapy, neurobiofeedback, "sensory-motor gym," nutritional counseling, homeschooling, ballet, drama, art, horseback riding, swimming, and karate? ("You're tearing my brain apart!" the young girl cried out on the day Trost tagged her, in the course of her second hour of vision therapy.)

However rarefied this world of specialized therapy may have been—"It's an expensive indulgence," a sidelined dad in the *New York* story dismissed it—psychiatric medication was, on the other hand, much more widely and deeply accessible, and medication use was the focus of a very widespread and passionate national conversation.

Ritalin use—which, we repeatedly read, had gone up 600 percent in the early 1990s, so that, by decade's end, fully 20 percent of white fifth-grade boys were on stimulant drugs for ostensible ADHD—had been the story for the better part of a decade. By 2004, however, the "Age of Ritalin," as *Time* magazine once dubbed it, had turned into a moment of major backlash, with much of the attention focused on SSRIs (selective serotonin reuptake inhibitors), the new class of antidepressants that had been hailed as something akin to miracle drugs—highly effective, with minimal side effects—in the late 1980s and early 1990s, after the introduction of Prozac.

Some very vocal critics from within the psychiatric profession were emerging to say that the drug industry had vastly underreported the potential dangers of the drugs, particularly for depressed teens, who were at greater risk of committing suicide because they had a higher rate of "suicidal ideation" when they were taking the new antidepressant medications. Much was made of reports that Eric Harris had been taking the SSRI Luvox in the weeks before he and Dylan Klebold shot up Columbine High School and committed suicide in 1999. (Harris said, however, in a videotaped message for posterity that he and Klebold made shortly before their rampage, that he had stopped taking the drug in order to let his anger flame.)

In March of 2004, a medical journal had revealed that the pharmaceutical company SmithKline Beecham (now GlaxoSmithKline) had withheld clinical findings from two studies that had shown that the antidepressant Paxil (paroxetine) was no more effective than placebo in treating adolescent depression and had also sought to manipulate data and suppress information that was "commercially unacceptable" regarding Paxil's use in children and teens.

Great Britain severely curtailed the use of antidepressants in children. The state of New York brought suit against Glaxo, charging that the company's manipulations and obfuscations amounted to fraud. Glaxo settled with New York State and agreed to pay $2.5 million and to publish all tests done on their drugs by 2005. The U.S. Food and Drug

Administration ordered all antidepressants to carry "black box" warnings saying they could increase the risk of suicidal thinking and behavior (called "suicidality") in children and adolescents. And doctors, worried about drugs like Prozac, encouraged by massive marketing efforts on the part of Big Pharma, and reassured by "thought leaders" in psychiatry who were actually in the pay of drugmakers, started more frequently to prescribe troubled children the much more powerful and dangerous antipsychotics instead.

Widespread public outrage followed revelations that even preschoolers as young as age two were now being given psychotropic drugs. Politicians got involved. The Clinton White House in 2000 had held a conference on young children's mental health and had begun a public health initiative aimed at reducing psychotropic medication use in the very young. Hearings were held on Capitol Hill, with experts like psychiatrist Peter Breggin called to testify that disorders like ADHD were, essentially, frauds perpetrated by leading psychiatrists, the National Institute of Mental Health, the drug companies, and parents working together to suppress the genius and creativity of disorderly children. "Children become diagnosed with ADHD when they are in conflict with the expectations or demands of parents and/or teachers," Breggin told members of Congress."The ADHD diagnosis is simply a list of the behaviors that most commonly cause conflict or disturbance in classrooms, especially those that require a high degree of conformity."

With parents alleging that schools were threatening to kick their children out of class unless they put them on medication, nine states passed or introduced legislation making it illegal for schools to talk to parents about medicating their kids. The Child Medication Safety Act, a bill protecting parents from being "coerced into administering a controlled substance," was passed by U.S. House of Representatives in 2004.

The medication of children became a particularly hot issue for the religious right after President Bush's New Freedom Commission on Mental Health in 2002 called for schools to play a bigger role in steering children toward mental health treatment and proposed national screening of kids for mental disorders. This fueled enormous Internet activity by conservative groups, evangelicals, Christian Scientists, and others fearful of government intrusion into family life and the forcible "drugging" of children.

Conservatives despaired that the growing diagnosis of ADHD was an attempt to "feminize" boys or neuter their natural boyishness. Many viewed the contemporary notion of mental illness as a brain disorder rather than a symptom of bad parenting as an assault on the idea of parental responsibility.

But the outrage over the medication of America's youth wasn't limited to conservatives, by any means. Fighting back against the drug companies, speaking out against the "sorcery" of psychiatrists, as *The Nation* columnist Alexander Cockburn once put it, was as much a part of being a self-respecting liberal, for many people, as despising George Bush and Dick Cheney. Like the Bush White House's cronies in the oil industry, drugmakers and psychiatrists—the "medicopharmaceutical industrial complex," as Richard DeGrandpre called them in his 2006 book, *The Cult of Pharmacology*—were seen as one more force of senseless order and soulless profiteering bearing down upon the American people.

Whether it came from the right, however, or the left, or the purely inane (Vince Vaughn, promoting his 2005 anti-Ritalin film, *Thumbsucker*, stressed his opposition to kids "sort of being doped up"), the basic premise of the story that emerged to explain why American childhood had taken on such a *Brave New World* aspect was always essentially the same: Children were being grossly overmedicated with dangerous and denaturing chemicals. The schools, the government, the drug companies, and psychiatrists had become a nefarious force bearing down on parents, corrupting childhood, and poisoning individual children's lives. And if there was anything truly going wrong with America's kids, it was their parents, the culture they were buying into, and the insane pressures of their pathological world.

I believed in this story unquestioningly when I began this book. I heard my friend's question about what I knew and how I knew it; it troubled me, vaguely. I worried afterward that a chill had come into our friendship (*Were we having "issues?"* I wondered). But the idea that her experience—her real-life journey through the world I was blithely describing—actually made some of my central views utterly ridiculous didn't dawn on me.

My certainty that kids with virtually no problems at all were being pathologized and pumped full of drugs was all but unshakable. As was the case in the burgeoning national discussion of children's mental health issues, that core belief went virtually unchallenged.

Because, on a gut level, it made sense.

After all, all around us was this crazy culture of parenting, full of competition and pressure and demands for kid-performance soaring to levels no one had ever seen before: First-grade work being done in kindergarten. College math in high school; high school math in seventh grade. And then there were these kids—all these kids—getting this alphabet soup of diagnoses that, before this insane period had begun, no one had ever heard of.

No one knew kids who were diagnosed with ADHD back in the 1950s or 1960s. No one knew kids who were "bipolar" back in the 1970s. You heard of retarded kids back then, sure—you knew of girls with eating disorders in the 1980s—you were yourself, perhaps, "depressed" in college (though you didn't get diagnosed, or take medication for it), but autism, Asperger's, PDD-NOS? Why were so many kids now being diagnosed with learning disabilities? And why were all these diagnoses happening so disproportionately in upper-middle-class communities?

It was easy, even natural, to put two and two together, and commentators of all types were doing it, all the time. "It may be a clue that the symptoms of many childhood psychiatric disorders seem to preclude schoolwork and attendance. Maybe the only problem with the kids is that they have been watching their own high-achieving parents, and they have seen where all that leads," the progressive author Barbara Ehrenreich wrote, for example, in *The New York Times*, reviewing journalist Paul Raeburn's heartbreaking account of dealing with his children's mental illnesses, *Acquainted with the Night*.

"What if at least some of what is being diagnosed in the child and adolescent population is not mental defect, neurochemical short-circuits, and the rest but, rather, the normal reactions of youngsters to the arguably inhuman rhythms of their days?" the conservative social critic Mary Eberstadt echoed, in her book, *Home-Alone America: The Hidden Toll of Day Care, Behavioral Drugs, and Other Parent Substitutes.*

It wasn't like I was out on a limb with my "social construction of disease." And yet.

And yet, I was having some issues.

In the winter of 2004, having spent much time scavenging, online and in local parenting papers, for professional parasites ("We do produce 'superhero' results," a nearby Learning Rx center promised of its "cognitive skills training and mental fitness" offerings) and for signs of neurotic parents looking to perfect their kids, I found a parent meeting in nearby Montgomery County that looked to be right up my alley.

It was called "Should I Worry . . . ?" and had been billed online as "A parent's perspective to help other parents figure out whether they should worry about their young child's behavior or emotional issues." It was sure to be, I was certain, a wellspring of good material.

I went to the meeting, which was in a church basement.

I introduced myself and took out my pen and notepad.

The evening began with a PowerPoint presentation. It was all acronyms and codes for navigating the public school system: IEP for individualized education program; Code 06—or ED—for emotional disturbance; RICA for Regional Institute for Children and Adolescents, the area's special school for emotionally disturbed children.

But the presentation couldn't really get very far, because every time the presenter stopped for questions, a seemingly bottomless well of emotion erupted. It wasn't parental anxiety, exactly, though there was plenty of that; it was sadness, and, in the parents who'd been living with the awareness of their kids' issues for years already and were there to help relative newcomers to their world, there was a kind of resignation.

Having arrived, jauntily expecting to hear about smart kids earning Bs instead of As, about boys too fidgety to sit through hours of seat work in kindergarten, or about girls melting down from the pressure of trying to please their impossible parents, I was profoundly confused.

There were no parents here trying to make their children superhuman. No one was talking of ways to up their kid's performance to gain admittance to the best private schools. They weren't looking to tinker around the edges of bad behavior or disappointing report cards. They were trying to figure out how to keep their kids in mainstream public schools and out of mental institutions. They were trying to educate themselves about navigating a system that would just as soon let their children drown. They'd come together because they felt utterly alone.

Alone with concerns like whether to call 911 when their teenage son was beating them up. Whether to push for an "LD" designation to keep a child out of a scary "ED" classroom.

One woman had seen a neighbor's kid "destroyed" by his time in an emotionally disturbed class. Another kid had "begged" to be taken out of the program, because he was afraid of the other kids. Worst of all was the prospect of having a child sent to RICA. No one wanted to go to RICA.

"Some of them go from RICA to jail," one mother said.

I heard of a little boy, "a seven-year-old who's a skinny toothpick," according to his mom, who, in a "major rage," had kicked a hole right through the bathroom wall.

And that was nothing.

Another mother described how any confrontation, even a minor correction on homework, would set off an explosion in her "tiny" nine-year-old adopted daughter from Russia. Her daughter's rage was "like a light switch," she said. "She'll push the table, break the pencils, jam the pencils into the table."

"When my child was in elementary school, it was manageable," said another mom. "There was some acting out but . . . unfortunately by middle school they're not so cute. One day, he took a friend's glasses and pounded them to smithereens. He just got worse and worse and they were about to throw him out of school."

There was a woman whose bipolar son's bouts of mania made him impossible to control. "Teachers, other parents ask, 'Why can't you discipline him?' " she related wryly. "There were times I wished I had a dart gun and could shoot him with a tranquilizer."

Another woman, with a sixteen-year-old son who refused to go to school, sympathized. "I can't get him there," she said.

A little girl whose brother was terrorizing the family was up in the middle of the night having panic attacks.

Some parents had been physically assaulted by their kids. Some were dealing with the guilt and heartbreak of seeing their children react badly—sometimes disastrously—to medication. One little boy, diagnosed with "severe attention issues," had started taking Adderall ("Behavior modification would have been fine, but my husband has ADD, and if my husband couldn't remember to do it, what good was behavior modification?") and, after six weeks of "poster boy" good behavior, ended up becoming psychotic.

Others were dealing with the mixed feelings of seeing their children do well with a lot of medication. One boy was taking Concerta for attention, Depakote for seizures, Xanax for anxiety, and Tenex "to bring him down a little bit," his mother said. "We had a hard time giving him medication. But he can't function without it."

"Now," she added, "he says, 'I love you.' "

"It was seven years before I heard my daughter say, 'I love you,' " the mother of the adopted Russian girl replied. "And when she does, I don't think she means it."

After the meeting, I drove off into the pitch-black night, in a pounding, punishing rain, feeling completely lost. For *Perfect Madness,* I had interviewed a lot of women about a lot of very personal, sometimes difficult feelings. But there was a lot of laughter, too. I had never experienced a level of pain like what I had just witnessed in that room.

"It was seven years before I heard my daughter say, 'I love you' . . . And when she does, I don't think she means it."

I cried on the way home that night, my tears further blurring the foggy windshield, making the near-invisible Beltway seem all the more like a long road to nowhere. I did not want to write this book.

The next morning, I woke up and looked over what I'd scribbled down over the course of the evening.

"THIS IS NOT WHAT I AM WRITING ABOUT," I scrawled across the top of my notepad. And then I put it away.

What was I writing about? What did I know?

I didn't know. As 2005 turned into 2006, I started trying to puzzle it out.

I wasn't writing about *real* mental illness like schizophrenia or bipolar disorder or whatever it was the kids whose parents were at the "Should I Worry?" group had, I at one point decided; I was only looking at the bogus "flavor-of-the-month" diagnoses, like ADHD and . . . bipolar disorder.

I was soon starting to despair. Sitting at my desk, trying to get a foothold on my topic, I started to feel more and more like I was sinking into quicksand, stuck in a dissolving hole of meaning whose walls collapsed every time I tried to climb out.

How did I know what was real and what was bogus? What was normal and what was disordered? What was pathology and what was parental projection?

I'd assembled a huge source list of experts whom I'd seen in the press denouncing our "crazy" culture, decrying overdiagnosis and overmedication, and dissecting the pathologies of family life in our time. Some of them, when I called them, jumped at the chance to get the word out on the fallacy of psychiatric diagnoses.

But others, given the bully pulpit, didn't quite run with it.

Child psychiatrist Alvin Rosenfeld, the coauthor, most recently, of *The Over-Scheduled Child: Avoiding the Hyper-Parenting Trap*, and a veteran of the faculties of Harvard and Stanford medical schools, had repeatedly warned, in an address to parents on "the overscheduled family," that hyperparenting could drive children to distraction: "This destructive force can weaken your marriage and get your beloved children overwhelmed, discouraged, and diagnosed as learning disabled, bipolar, ADD, anxious and depressed."

But he politely demurred as I ranted about the falsity of the ADHD diagnosis and the inappropriateness of medication. "That certainly hasn't been my experience," he said.

Psychologist and *The Blessing of a Skinned Knee* author Wendy Mogel, another critic of perfectionistic high-stress parenting, urged "compassion" over "finger-wagging."

"One of the main things I'm struck with every single day is the enormous amount of love that parents have for their children," said Dana Kornfeld, a popular D.C.-area pediatrician who, like most children's primary-care providers, treats many patients with emotional and behavioral issues. "Literally forty times a day I see how intensely parents, especially mothers, love their kids and worry about their kids. It's not pathological," she insisted.

This charge—however veiled—of being harsh, of being unsympathetic and overly judgmental, wasn't necessarily new to me. By this time, *Perfect*

Madness had been published, and of all the many criticisms of it, the ones that had most stuck in my mind, and most profoundly gotten under my skin, were the ones that concerned blind spots in my ability to empathize with other parents. They troubled me precisely because they really did point to blind spots—I hadn't seen those particular criticisms coming, and I couldn't quite understand them.

A local mother, whose son had nearly died in her arms of anaphylactic shock after ingesting peanuts, hadn't appreciated my use of peanut allergy as a metaphor for the effects of excessive parental worry. Ellen Galinksy, president and cofounder of Families and Work Institute, and a woman I greatly admire, had suggested that my arguments in support of families could have been stronger, had I been capable of greater empathy toward individual parents. "What you have to remember," she said, "is that most parents just want the best for their children, and are doing the best they can."

In a book talk I would give after *Perfect Madness* came out, I had a line that I thought was powerful and true: "We all have our worries and our own particular magical weapons with which we think we can get some kind of control over our world and make the things we most worry about come out all right. . . . For some, it's therapy—this therapy and that therapy and on and on until *some therapy*, finally, will provide the silver bullet that will make the most intractable-seeming problems go away." I'd never understood why some parents recoiled, as though hit by an electric shock, when I delivered it. Why some looked down, why others looked so angry.

Plenty of people were saying the same thing as me. Some (though not so many, once I scratched the surface of reporting) were mental health professionals. Others were Christian conservatives. Or proxies for the Church of Scientology, whose Citizens Committee on Human Rights had just opened a museum in Hollywood.

It was called Psychiatry: An Industry of Death.

A number of the experts whose names and previously published quotes I'd originally collected to build up my research turned out to be kind of . . . "out there." Bethesda psychiatrist Peter Breggin, for example, a frequent expert witness in a series of lawsuits regarding Ritalin in the late 1990s, had been either excluded from testifying or discredited by judges. ("Dr. Breggin's observations are totally without credibility. I can almost declare him, I guess from statements that floor me, to say he's a fraud or at least approaching that . . . . He's untrained. He's a member of no hospital staff. He has not since medical school participated in any studies to support his conclusions except maybe one. . . . I can't place any credence or credibility in what he has to recommend in this case," Judge James W. Rice of the Milwaukee County Circuit Court had declared in *Schellinger v. Schellinger,* in 1997.)

This all gave me pause. Was I really on the right track? Ideologically, philosophically, was I running with the right crowd?

Why was I, like the nutty Tom Cruise and utterly inarticulate CCHR proxy Juliette Lewis, ready to believe the absolute worst of psychiatry and psychiatrists? *How did I know*—as I unquestioningly had assumed I did—that they were rushing to drug kids for the sake of high performance and conformity, colluding with parents eager to get their kids on the Harvard track as early as possible?

Where had these certainties come from?

The answer to that question didn't come to me until the fall of 2006, by which time the manuscript for this book was officially one year past due. I was sitting in our local coffeehouse, as I often did in those days, reading David Healy's *The Creation of Psychopharmacology.*

Healy, a professor of psychiatry and director of the North Wales Department of Psychological Medicine at Cardiff University, was one of the first and most vocal critics of the risks and limitations of using SSRIs to treat depression. In the late 1990s, he'd been an unwelcome voice raising the specter of suicide risks. In his 2004 book, *Let Them Eat Prozac,* he'd blasted the ties between the pharmaceutical industry and the psychiatric establishment, even arguing that it was the advent of the SSRIs, notably Prozac, that had actually *created* modern depression. (That is to say: the categorization of levels of suffering that previously would have passed under the radar as chemically treatable conditions.) He was an outsider, but he was also a compelling writer who had the grudging respect of many within the psychiatric establishment.

A history of psychopharmacology should have been dry reading. But Healy's wasn't, for me. Reading it turned out to be a scales-falling-from-the-eyes experience.

First came the surprise of learning, when I got up to the discovery of chlorpromazine, which was launched in the United States in 1954 as Thorazine, and proved to be the first schizophrenia treatment that worked, that psychiatrists had joyfully celebrated the drug because they saw it as "liberating patients."

Psychiatrists celebrating liberation? This was a new one.

But the sentence that really did me in, the one that, in an instant, brought the whole intellectual edifice of this book crumbling at my feet, was a quote from Jean-Paul Sartre. It was a line from a foreword he'd written to the Scottish psychiatrist R. D. Laing's 1967 book, *The Politics of Experience*: *"Mental illness is the revolt that the free organism in its total entity invents in order to live in an unbearable situation."*

Maybe you're laughing now. Maybe you're confused. Wasn't Sartre simply saying what I'd been thinking all along?

Well, yes, of course. And that was the whole problem.

Sartre, Laing, the French philosopher Michel Foucault—and the whole group of radical writers and thinkers who ultimately came to form the antipsychiatry movement—they'd all believed that psychiatric symptoms were symbolic expressions of social pathology. That psychiatrists were storm troopers for the forces of hegemonic social conformity. That psychiatric patients weren't sick; they were just "canaries in the coal mine" for our sick society.

Healy devoted a whole section of his book to the antipsychiatry movement. After reading it, I let the book drop next to my long-cold coffee. I closed my eyes in dismay.

Once upon a time, as a teenager with intellectual pretensions, I'd idolized Jean-Paul Sartre.

Once upon a time, like many lefty literature students in the 1980s, I'd, with great seriousness and pride of purpose, read Michel Foucault. And Roland Barthes and Jacques Derrida—that whole generation of sixties-era French intellectuals, who, by the Reagan eighties, were chiefly being read in American humanities departments, where their once-radicalism seemed fresh and subversive, and new.

They'd certainly seemed that way to me. "Theory"—as we referred to the work of the kinds of thinkers I mentioned above—taught that nothing had any intrinsic meaning. Male/female, gay/straight, good/evil, all was just language, "discourse," power relations, socially constructed systems of signification designed to lock you in. For a nineteen-year-old in the full throes of a somewhat delayed adolescent rebellion, this felt revolutionary. Utterly thought-liberating. A wonderful way to upend everything I'd ever been told about gender, identity, and normality.

Perhaps this all sounds silly to you now. It sounds silly to me. But back then, it was dead serious. "Theory" was like religion for me—until, one day, it wasn't. That is to say, until I went to graduate school and somehow, en route to a never-finished Ph.D., sort of outgrew it. Sitting in literature seminars with professors who seemed to be forever dreaming of escape, I grew disenchanted with all the sterile abstraction. I came to feel that some things did have meaning, that there was a distinction between what was real and what was "discourse." I decided that I wanted to dwell and work in the world of reality. I grew up.

Or so I thought.

Sitting there in the coffeehouse, finding my current thoughts echoed so exactly in the antipsychiatry thinkers of the 1960s, I wondered if I'd really grown up, intellectually, at all.

Was I really doing my own thinking?

Was I really engaging with reality?

Did I really want to be operating on this level?

There are many great things that grew out of the social rebellions of the 1960s. The lefty intellectual reflex of antipsychiatry—which, the University of Toronto medical historian Edward Shorter has noted, has become nothing less than a "new orthodoxy" among academics in America—is not necessarily one of them. "To an extent unimaginable for other areas of the history of medicine, zealot-researchers have seized the history of psychiatry to illustrate how their pet bugaboos—be they capitalism, patriarchy, or psychiatry itself—have converted protest into illness, locking into asylums those who otherwise would be challenging the established order," he wrote in his 1997 book, *A History of Psychiatry: From the Era of the Asylum to the Age of Prozac.* "Although these trendy notions have attained great currency among intellectuals, they are incorrect, in that they do not correspond to what actually happened."

Of course, there was much about the practices of the American psychiatric profession in the mid-twentieth century that was wrong. The profession was rife with misogyny, homophobia, and racism. Medication, even the barbarity of lobotomy was sometimes used punitively, and patients in state hospitals often received grossly inadequate, shamefully neglectful care. Like the society around it, psychiatry absolutely needed to change.

Yet what the antipsychiatry movement ultimately brought about in the United States—the deinstitutionalization of hundreds of thousands of mental patients, many of whom ended up living, and dying, on the streets—was a humanitarian disaster. And its intellectual legacy, which lives on not only in academia but also throughout our cultural mainstream, has been in many ways extremely destructive. It has led us to romanticize illnesses like depression and anxiety, even autism and schizophrenia, as free and "authentic" ways of being.

At best, this way of thinking is foolish. At worst, it is inhuman and cruel.

I realized, that day in the coffeehouse, that what I'd be trying to do—"read" the culture, deconstruct kids' diagnoses by analyzing them symbolically—was no different from when, in college, I'd read Derrida's analysis of Aristotle without ever having read Aristotle. I was erecting a whole intellectual edifice upon ignorance.

I didn't want to do it anymore.

What was the antidote? To get my facts straight. To put together a story that wasn't filled with holes and intellectual contradictions. To write something that would establish some kind of baseline reality from which a truly productive discussion of children's mental health issues could take place.

What that first meant was defining that reality: How many kids really had mental health issues? What was the nature of those issues, and were they really epidemic? Why did they appear to be so greatly on the rise? Were they real? Were parents pushing kids into pseudomadness? Why were parents willing to "drug" their kids? How did they feel about it? How did they arrive at that point? What were their lives like?

It was, I decided, dusting off the "Should I Worry?" notes, time to listen and learn. And so, in 2007—two years after my book was actually due—I set out to engage with my subject. I interviewed as many psychiatrists, psychologists, and parents of children with mental health issues as time permitted. The parents, about sixty in all, had children with autism, Asperger's, ADHD, anxiety disorders, OCD, bipolar disorder, dyspraxia, dyslexia, and sensory integration issues—in short, the range of disorders that I had once dismissed as "fashionable maladies." (And that I will, from here on, refer to as "mental disorders," "mental health disorders," "mental health issues," or "mental illnesses.")*

These parents had suffered enormously. They weren't living with symbolic representations of social pathologies. They were living with children who wrote themselves off as stupid at age five. Or threatened suicide at seven. Or were for years the butt of bullies' jokes and harassment because they were too spaced-out socially to clue into what their "friends" were really up to.

They were parents who laughed at the idea people had that they were trying to create "perfect" children. They had children who, left untreated, pretty much couldn't function at all.

I found that, rather than pushing to get their kids diagnosed, these parents had wanted nothing more than for their kids to be "normal." That rather than rushing to "drug" their kids, the parents had most frequently done everything they could to avoid giving their children medication.

Many had started out having their concerns for their children dismissed by pediatricians. Many had received poor quality psychiatric care. Yet the story that emerged from that poor care wasn't one, overall, of overdiagnosis and overmedication, but, rather, of shoddy diagnosis and poorly administered medical care. Add to that a big dose of stigma and you get, in a nutshell, the state of most children's mental health care in America.

The truth is, despite all we read about parents who seek to protect

---

* In 1999, the U.S. Surgeon General defined children's "mental disorders" as "serious deviations from expected cognitive, social, and emotional development." The National Institute of Mental Health, which defines as its purview "the evolving science of brain, behavior and experience," categorizes such disorders of childhood, plus post-traumatic stress disorder and schizophrenia, simply as "mental illness." The commonality of them all is that they involve some kind of brain dysfunction or abnormality of brain development. For most people, I think, "mental illness" brings to mind mood and thought disorders like manic-depression and schizophrenia only. Perhaps that has to change. At any rate, in the interest of avoiding an unbearable degree of repetition, I will be using the phrases "mental disorders," "mental health disorders," "mental health issues," and "mental illness" interchangeably here.

their kids from any and all mental anguish, the vast majority of kids in America who have real mental health needs don't get any help.

They don't get it because there isn't money to pay for it and because there's a shortage of practitioners to provide it. And they don't get it because of the pervasiveness of views like my former certitudes: the doubt that mental health problems are real, the aspersion cast on parents of children with problems, the confusion over what mental health disorders actually are, the tendency to conflate mental illness with bad behavior, and to see children symbolically—as the designated patients in a culture we all can agree is pathological—instead of as real people.

That web of belief—let's call it the "naysayer" position, as I have seen others do—is the new face of mental health stigma in our time. It is voiced as concern, as a desire to save children, as a wish to give childhood back to kids, but what it really is, most of the time, is prejudice. And it's a poison.

People who share the views I used to espouse don't see themselves as prejudiced. They believe they are raising their voices in protest of a world that's gone mad, and, in particular, providing necessary push back against a pharmaceutical industry that's grown way too powerful, with the collusion of our government and far too many research scientists and clinical practitioners.

I want to say here as strongly as I can that I agree that many aspects of today's world of childhood are toxic and that I deplore both the irresponsible marketing practices of Big Pharma and the failure of our government and research institutions to stand up against it. I think that individual psychiatrists who have enriched themselves by turning into shadow employees of drug companies have dealt their profession a terrible blow, from which it will take a great deal of time—and reform—to recover. That said, I also fiercely believe that the social climate of family life, the machinations of the pharmaceutical industry, and the lives of children and parents dealing with mental health issues have to be viewed as separate phenomena. Not because they aren't interconnected, but because if you let your feelings about industry and society cloud your vision of parents and children, you run the risk of not seeing them at all.

We can hate the world of our current creation—the rushed, pressured, competitive, cutthroat realm of middle- and upper-middle-class American childhood—without writing off the children in it. We can dislike certain trends in contemporary parenting without vilifying parents to the point where we can't see when they're in pain or need help. And we must—if we're going to make any progress in understanding the complexities of children's mental health issues in our day.

Those parents you see, going from doctor to doctor and trying pill after pill? They're scared. They need help. And so do their kids.

· 2 ·

Seeing Is Believing

"If I didn't believe in it, I wouldn't see it."

Rosalie Greenberg, professor of clinical psychiatry at Columbia University, on the existence of bipolar disorder in young children

My father struggled terribly with anxiety. I have other family members who suffer from mental illness as well—ADHD, bipolar disorder, depression, mostly.

And if I think about the extended family, and look at the evolution of individual relatives' lives over the decades, a pattern is very clear. People who have gotten good treatment have gotten better—or at least have had some ability to live some semblance of the lives they were meant to have. People who have not gotten treatment have gotten stuck. Stuck professionally, stuck emotionally, isolated within their illnesses and cursed with a constant, pained awareness of what their lives could have been.

I knew much of this when I was going into this book. I knew, at least, that I had lost a father to untreated mental illness. Yet none of this knowledge kept me from viewing the business of children's mental health diagnoses and treatments as a scam. None of it kept me from doubting the reality of children's psychiatric diagnoses and imputing the worst possible motivations to the child psychiatrists who treated them. None of it—not even the very dramatic experience of having watched people close to me brought back to life with the use of antidepressant medications—led me to doubt my belief that to give kids drugs was a scandal: dangerous, irresponsible, and unnecessary. And none of it kept me from thinking that there had to be, metaphorically at least, something in the water creating all the weird, new "issues" in kids that I was reading about all the time.

I was not alone in these beliefs. Neither was I alone in the experience of having witnessed mental illness close up. I couldn't have been: At least 25 percent of American adults in any given year suffer to some degree from a mental disorder. About half of those people are severely affected enough to need treatment. Six percent are so impaired that they attempt suicide or have substantial limitations to their daily functioning.

That's a lot of people. There are also a lot of people right now taking psychotropic medication: 33 million were prescribed at least one psychiatric drug in 2004.

Given that so many people do have mental health issues, and do take medication, acknowledging both the reality of their suffering and the belief that there is an at least partial biological basis for that suffering; given that, as a society, we claim to applaud people for facing up to their mental health issues and dealing with them, why is there such universal condemnation for extending similar treatment to kids?

Why is it so hard to acknowledge that children's mental disorders also are common, impairing, at least in part genetic, and real?

Why is there so much resistance to the idea that a fair number of children—a small and yet not inconsequential percentage—require psychiatric treatment, and medication in particular?

Why do we accept that, say, a condition like diabetes has a genetic component, shows up in childhood, and should be treated as early as possible, but resist extending this same sort of logic to mental illness?

Why, in short, is there such incredible cognitive dissonance?

In my own case, I can now see that my muddled thinking came in large part from simple prejudice—against psychiatrists, and against parents. It was also partly ignorance: an unawareness that more than half, and perhaps as many as two-thirds of the people who suffer from mental illness as adults began to have symptoms as children. And it was partly, at base, because the very idea that children could have mental health issues other than essentially normal responses to bad parenting was so very alien to me.

I was not alone, once again, in holding such views. For most people, the notion that many kids can have psychiatric issues that go beyond the normal developmental hiccups of growing up is very new and very suspect.

After all, when my generation of parents was growing up, in the late 1950s or 1960s, or even the 1970s, you never saw kids on meds. No one, for that matter, knew kids who had ADHD, or bipolar disorder, or Asperger's.

Or so it seemed.

"I always had tutors. I thought I was dumb. People thought I was lazy. I thought I was lazy," a Washington, D.C., woman, eyes downcast, voice tremulous, told me and a roomful of mothers of kids with learning disabilities, anxiety disorders, dyspraxia, autism, and ADHD, one beautiful spring day in 2007. "I missed a whole lot. I'd just get papers back with zeros. With a really mean, Victorian-age teacher. Everyone would know when your eyes would be tearing up, and it was humiliating."

These mothers knew one another from soccer fields and from playgrounds. They'd come together on that morning, as they did every so often, to talk about their kids and to compare notes on doctors, therapies, meds, and schools. With me there that day, each was telling the story of the journey she'd made in the course of figuring out that her son or daughter had "issues."

For the woman in question, a former lawyer who'd struggled mightily from middle school through law school and was now a stay-at-home mom, learning that her daughters had the inattentive subtype of ADHD had been like lifting a veil. It got to the root of some very basic mysteries at the center of her own life: Why had she had such a hard time in school? Why had she always felt so bad about herself? Why had she been swamped with such anxiety during the first visit to her daughters' school, the same Catholic school that she had attended as a girl?

The sight of the classrooms had brought back a sick-to-the-stomach feeling of dread.

"You know you're not stupid, but everything in your world makes you doubt that about yourself," she remembered. "Every interaction you have. You don't quite get it socially. You have people telling you you're lazy and why don't you just work harder. But you yourself know that you're thinking creatively. You have some really amazing ideas but they can't come out. It's horrible. It eats at your very core of self-esteem."

When her daughters began having trouble in school and were diagnosed with ADHD, the mother started reading up on the ways the disorder expresses itself in girls. And the story of her own life took on new meaning: "I was just crying, reading," she told the assembled moms. "It was the revelation of . . . you're not stupid."

If you want to find people who can attest to the fact that in the past children did, rather commonly, have mental health issues, you need look no further than the parents of today's diagnosed kids. For many of them experienced firsthand in their youth the kinds of struggles that their children are now going through.

They didn't have a label for their problems then. They couldn't name them or even articulate the nature of their experience.

"I was just in a fog," a Boston-area mother of a depressed eight-year-old boy recalled of her own school years lived under a cloud of depression. "It went through phases. It came in bouts. I don't remember learning anything in school."

Teachers, parents, other children provided labels for these kids. Things like "dumb." "Lazy." "Bad." "Weird."

The labels generally weren't very productive.

"When I was a kid, the diagnoses were 'smart' or 'stupid.' The treatments were try harder or get spanked," Boston-area psychiatrist Edward M. Hallowell, whose 1994 *Driven to Distraction* (coauthored with John J. Ratey) helped put attention deficit disorder on the cultural map, remarked of his own experience of growing up with dyslexia and ADHD in the 1950s and early 1960s.

"My sibling made it to fifth grade before anyone noticed he couldn't read," a woman at the "Should I Worry?" meeting in Maryland recalled of her brother, who, forty years earlier, used to turn over desks and smash up classrooms. "He was what was called a 'juvenile delinquent' at the time."

The self-labeling—and self-punishing—experienced by kids who today would be diagnosed with "issues" could be even worse.

"In school I was bright, I knew I was, but I always heard things like you don't try hard enough," another D.C. mother, who learned she had ADHD and dyslexia after her son was diagnosed with learning issues, said in a phone interview. "I was always humiliated. I had a teacher who placed us in the classroom in math according to our grades and I was always in the back of the room. All my friends were these A students who got it. You're not like that and you see yourself drifting because you're not able to keep up in their classes. At the end of every school year I'd be beating up on myself, saying, 'You've got to get organized and you're going to make it,' and the new school year would start and it would take off so fast and I'd be lost, and I'd be beating up on myself all over again."

Children like these weren't diagnosed a generation ago. Many, if not most, of the diagnoses common today simply did not exist then. Or they were defined very differently, so narrowly, perhaps, as to draw in just a tiny number of kids. And they only drew in those kids if parents thought to take their children in to see a psychiatrist, which most parents didn't do. All that has changed, and change has come very rapidly.

Since the early 1990s, the number of children receiving diagnoses of mental health disorders has tripled. This vast increase in diagnosis has fed enormous skepticism. "If children cough after exercising, they have asthma; if they have trouble reading, they are dyslexic; if they are unhappy, they are depressed; and if they alternate between unhappiness and liveliness, they have bipolar disorder," is how H. Gilbert Welch, Lisa Schwartz, and Steven Woloshin, physician-researchers affiliated with the White River Junction Outcomes Group, put it in *The New York Times* in January 2007.

The increase has also fed talk of "epidemics"—higher than could normally be expected outbreaks of autism, depression, anxiety, and ADHD, most notably. "Something's rotten in the state of our children's mental health," warned UPI in 2006. "Mind-boggling trends are snaking their way into the record books, rattling the nation with reams of reports of nearly 14 million youngsters, some of them barely out of diapers, beset by a plethora of psychiatric disturbances."

The idea that these kids with psychiatric issues have somehow suddenly sprung up from nowhere is a mainstay of the naysayer position.

Yet it just isn't true that kids didn't have mental health issues before. The problems existed, even if the diagnoses didn't. Plenty of adults remember having them. In 2005, in fact, a major national survey found that fully half of the adults with mental health disorders recalled starting to suffer from their symptoms by the time they were fourteen. The median age of onset for anxiety and "impulse control disorders" was age eleven.

Daniel Pine, a specialist in mood and anxiety disorders at the National Institute of Mental Health, believes that this 50 percent number is low. About two-thirds of adults who suffer from mental illness had at least some antecedents in childhood, he says. "If you look at affected adults between the ages of twenty and forty who have depression," for example, he told me, "you would find about 60 percent of them, if you had seen them as kids, would have had a clearly identifiable mental health problem."

Adding on to this, I'd like to suggest the idea that if *today's* doctors could have looked at yesterday's children, they would undoubtedly have seen "clearly identifiable" mental health problems. But yesterday's doctors—and parents, schools, and society at large—looked at children very differently. If children had problems like ADHD, depression, or dyslexia then, no one had the eyes to see them. Or the words—or even the concepts—to provide many of the diagnoses so common today.

The idea that children can suffer from mental illness isn't new. Although it was not until the 1930s that child psychiatry emerged as a unique specialty, medical references to children's "passions of the mind" date as far back as 1789. In 1844, the German psychiatrist Heinrich Hoffmann provided the first known description of what would today be called ADHD in a poem titled, "The Story of Fidgety Phil": *He turns/And churns/He wiggles/And jiggles/Here and there on the chair/Phil, these twists I cannot bear.*

Toward the end of the nineteenth century, Emil Kraepelin, the German clinician and researcher commonly referred to as the "father of modern psychiatry" for his biologically oriented classification system of mental disorders, reported seeing depression, hallucinatory schizophrenia, "mental explosiveness," and suicide in young patients, and estimated manic depression to occur in .5 percent of prepubescent children. Asylum psychiatrists generally, by the turn of the twentieth century, had come to believe that all forms of "insanity" existed in children as well as in adults.

But in the period when most of today's adults were growing up, the prevailing vision was very different. It was the period of Freudian hegemony in American psychiatry.

The Freudians believed that depression could not show up in children until they hit puberty, because their egos were not well-enough developed to be vulnerable to such troubles. They similarly believed that manic depression, as bipolar disorder was previously called, could emerge only in the late teens or in early adulthood. Hyperactive kids were known, until 1968, as having "minimal brain dysfunction," a label derived from early-twentieth-century doctors' observations that children with no known neurological disease could exhibit the kind of hyperactivity previously seen in children with encephalitis. After 1968, they were diagnosed with "hyperkinetic reaction of childhood or adolescence."

There weren't many standard, agreed-upon psychiatric diagnoses for children in the period in which psychoanalysis held sway. In the *Diagnostic and Statistical Manual* of 1952, the American Psychiatric Association's first attempt to create a standardized classification system of mental disorders, there were only four: "schizophrenic reaction, childhood type," and, in a section on Transient Situational Personality Disorders, "adjustment reactions" of infancy, childhood, and adolescence. The adjustment reactions of childhood were further broken down into subcategories for "habit disturbance"—things like nail-biting, thumb-sucking, masturbation, and tantrums; "conduct disturbance"—stealing, destructiveness, cruelty, sexual offenses, use of alcohol; and "neurotic traits," which were things like tics, stammering, "overactivity," and phobias.

The second edition of the *DSM*, published in 1968, had a separate section for Behavior Disorders of Childhood and Adolescence. These, the authors noted, were problems more "stable, internalized, and resistant to treatment" than those that could be called mere issues of life adjustment. Here, for the first time, was hyperkinetic reaction of childhood or adolescence—comprised of "overactivity, restlessness, distractibility and short attention span." There was "withdrawing reaction," characterized by seclusiveness, detachment, sensitivity, shyness, and a "general inability to form close interpersonal relationships." There was "overanxious reaction," in which the "patient tends to be immature, self-conscious, grossly lacking in self-confidence, conforming, inhibited, dutiful, approval-seeking and apprehensive in new situations and unfamiliar surroundings." There was "unsocialized aggressive reaction," diagnosed in children who showed "hostile disobedience, quarrelsomeness, physical and verbal aggressiveness, vengefulness and destructiveness," and there was "runaway reaction," which, as the name implies, applied to children who ran away from home.

Reading the descriptions of yesterday's disorders, it becomes more difficult to maintain the view that today's psychiatrists uniquely pathologize children. There certainly was a notion of what was normal or abnormal a generation ago (or perhaps better put: what was adapative or maladaptive). What was greatly different then— beyond the nomenclature—is that children's problems that would today be seen at least in part as inborn and brain-based, were viewed solely in the early *DSMs* as reactions to the environment. (Even "learning disturbance" is characterized, in *DSM-I*, as a "special symptom reaction" under the rubric of Personality Disorders.)

The more banal, transient disorders were reactions to life events—the birth of a sibling, difficulties in school—but the more lasting problems were reactions to bad parents. The "schizophrenogenic mother," in particular, was believed to be at the root of most childhood mental disorders. She could make her child psychotic by being both cold and rejecting and demanding and controlling all at once. She could make her child autistic ("autistic, atypical and withdrawn behavior" being a symptom of childhood schizophrenia) by refusing him her love, or simply failing to provide the love he needed in just the right way.

For very sick children, the standard treatment, in Freudian times, was a "parentectomy"—removal of the offending parent from a child's life by transferring the child into institutional care. Children we'd now call autistic were routinely institutionalized in the postwar years. Far less afflicted children were sent away, too, if their parents could be talked into it.

In her 2003 book, *Laughing Allegra,* Anne Ford, a great-granddaughter of Henry Ford, recalls how in the mid-1970s she was urged to send her young child, who had severe learning issues at a time when the term "learning disability" was not yet in widespread use, far away. Ford went from specialist to specialist in Manhattan, using all her family connections and considerable resources, until finally she ended up in the office of "one of the most respected pediatric psychiatrists in the city," who told her that her five-year-old daughter, Allegra, was "borderline retarded" and ought to be sent to an institution—outside of London. "I think you are making the problem worse," he said. "It really would be best if she was taken away from you." (Thanks to her perseverance—and substantial funds—Ford was able to avoid such extreme measures. She eventually found a specialized private school for her daughter. Allegra ultimately went to college, in a special program for adults with learning disabilities, and found work as a teacher's aide in Head Start.)

In the postwar period in America, children who were sent away for emotional or behavioral problems often stayed away for years. They didn't have to be dangerous or psychotic for this to happen. Sometimes, they were just intractably difficult.

Such, at least, was the case for Mindy Lewis, a New York writer and artist who, in 1967, at the age of fifteen, was sent for twenty-seven months to the New York State Psychiatric Institute at Columbia-Presbyterian Medical Center.

The symptoms of disorder that brought her there: "using marijuana . . . staying away from home, lying about her whereabouts, and being truant from school," her hospital records indicate.

Her diagnosis: "Acute schizophrenic reaction with marked premorbid hysterical features." Her treatment: Thorazine.

When I began this book and started out reading and talking to experts, generally nonpsychiatrists who were critical of the way children's mental health care is practiced today and sympathetic to my early vision of my topic, I expected to encounter stories of how things were done better in the past. I thought people would say that, a generation or so ago, children's mental health specialists were more rational, more cautious, more humanistic. But I heard no such nostalgia. Psychologist Wendy Mogel recalled teenagers, as late as the 1980s, being put in the hospital "for six months if they didn't get along with their stepmother."

"When I entered the field in the very early eighties," she said, "we had no terms for learning disabilities. We had one little phrase, minimal brain dysfunction, that's all we knew. And pervasive developmental delay came out a little bit later. We had no medications for adolescents except Thorazine. The 'schizophrenogenic mother' was completely scapegoated. . . . And let's say there was a kid who had a learning disability in adolescence; nobody would notice that because we were all so busy with the legacy of heritage, of family dysfunction passed on through the generations."

Northern California behavioral pediatrician Larry Diller, one of the most vocal critics of child psychiatry today, recalled how, in medical school in the 1970s, he'd been taught that a ten-year-old boy's problem with bed-wetting "stemmed from watching his parents perform the sex act." Diller's instructor would hear of no treatment other than play therapy "to work through the trauma." When Diller proposed treating the boy with behavioral techniques, which then, as now, had been proven to be highly effective, he nearly failed the class.

The psychiatrists I interviewed were even more categorical in their rejection of the Freudian past. Having trained on the pediatric psych wards of the 1960s, 1970s, and 1980s, they had memories of children in restraints, in seclusion rooms, on locked units. As late as the 1980s, they remembered children (commonly diagnosed by then with "conduct disorders" rather than schizophrenia), zonked out on the antipsychotics Thorazine and Haldol or on the mood-stabilizer lithium, not because the kids were delusional or bipolar, but because the drugs were sedating, the kids were out of control, and there really wasn't much of anything else to do. The drugs brought the children under control. They also made their bodies rigid, their movements stiff or shaky; sometimes their limbs flailed, uncontrollably.

Dr. Harold Koplewicz, director of the New York University Child Study Center and author of the 1996 book *It's Nobody's Fault: New Hope and Help for Difficult Children and Their Parents*, recalled an environment in which parents were made to feel terrible shame, child psychiatrists did their work without the benefit of a large body of research, diagnoses were makeshift and vague, and children's treatment could drag on fruitlessly for months, even years. "Back in those days, we weren't rigorous about diagnosis. You'd spend sessions and sessions playing with the kid, in a very slow process of information-gathering, so the kids who were 'in treatment' were going for a long time without a diagnosis," he told me. "It was mysterious. It was confusing. Parents didn't understand what was going on. It was more diffuse and there was somehow an implication that the doctor knew some secret and couldn't share it with you as a parent. No one told that your kid went to a therapist. If you saw someone, the idea was that your kid was crazy. The big C."

The years-long hospitalizations that so many children were put through, Dr. David Shaffer, chief of the Division of Child and Adolescent Psychiatry at Columbia University Medical Center, told me, often ended up doing at least as much harm as good. The psych wards, he said, where children lived and attended school—such as it was—were "somewhat deprived environments."

> *"The patients were getting a second-rate education, they were spending their time with children with problems, they had almost no contact with*

their parents. There was the notion that patients were experiencing some kind of treatment but the theories of what they were treating were so poorly developed. People didn't have any very good ideas of what psychotherapy could consist of. Child psychoanalysis was a pretty sleepy thing. It would often involve so-called play therapy, with occasional interpretations which I think were often very difficult for a child to understand and no systematic evaluations to see if anyone was getting better."

Dr. Shaffer came to Columbia in the 1970s, after training at the Maudsley Hospital in London. "When I first came here, one of the first things I did," he said, "was close down our young children's ward."

In the late 1980s and 1990s, children's psych wards around the country started closing. Adult psychiatric hospitals did, too. Largely, this was driven by economics: Insurance companies would no longer pay for long-term care. But money wasn't the only factor driving the change.

A rebellion against Freudianism, a push to ground American psychiatry in the study of neurobiology, brain chemistry, and genetics, had been growing in pockets of American academia since the late 1940s, and by the 1980s, it had reached critical mass. Many doctors now believed that psychoanalysis simply didn't work for patients other than mildly affected "neurotics" (who, it appeared, felt better over time no matter what you did with them).

There was a growing interest in using medication to fight severe mental illness, which psychoanalysis had been particularly ineffective in treating. The discovery of chlorpromazine (marketed in the United States in 1954 as Thorazine), had been a watershed moment in psychiatry; for the first time there was a treatment that worked for psychotics. The discovery of imipramine, the first medication marketed specifically as an antidepressant (as Tofranil, in 1958), was similarly epoch-making. Lithium, recognized for its psychotropic effects in the late 1940s, but not marketed in the United States until 1970 because of resistance from the psychoanalytic establishment, was the first treatment to put a cap on mania. This was world-changing stuff.

In 1980, the so-called "biological" psychiatrists' dominance over the profession was made official when the American Psychiatric Association published the third edition of its diagnostic "bible," the *Diagnostic and Statistical Manual of Mental Disorders*. The *DSM-III* was purged of Freudian terminology like "neurosis" and "hysteria" and brought into being the symptom-based system of disorder classification known to us today. Attention Deficit Disorder now got its name, conceived not as a "reaction" to anything, but as a constellation of symptoms that were presumed to have an organic cause.

The psychoanalytic vision of children's mental health ostensibly came to an end at this time. Yet change wasn't immediate, and the attitude shift embodied within the *DSM-III* was far from universal. It had not, for example, trickled down to the psychiatric clinic where Harold Koplewicz saw his first patient as a young psychiatrist on the cusp of all this change, in 1980.

The patient was a twelve-year-old boy who was acting out and failing in school. The boy had a working mother, a missing testicle due to an early cancer, and (relevantly) the pattern of learning and behavioral problems that the *DSM-III* had just officially labeled ADD.

"If you looked at the school records, you saw he couldn't sit still, he couldn't focus," Koplewicz told me. "But all his problems were blamed on the fact that his parents were divorced, and he'd been born with cancer and had had a testicle removed. All the other doctors were focusing on that and on the fact that his father had been a taxi driver, then had been bored with being a taxi driver and with the gas shortage had become a jockey. I was just as focused as everyone else on the fact that he felt damaged by the surgery and his father was a failure and his mother was the breadwinner—'castrating.' It took me months to come up with a diagnosis."

Koplewicz eventually suggested that the boy had ADD and recommended putting him on Ritalin. "The father said no: 'You're not putting my kid on drugs,'" he recalled. "So it was another year. Things started falling apart academically in middle school. It's so disorganizing, he was barely holding it together, failing. The mother decided to let him be put on meds, in spite of the father."

A year later, the boy invited Koplewicz to his bar mitzvah. He asked him to pretend to be the family veterinarian. But at the reception, "He went and introduced me to everyone as 'my friend,'" Koplewicz said.

The decline of Freudianism did not translate, early on, into greatly increased drug treatments for kids. It wasn't until the late 1980s and early 1990s that psychiatrists started prescribing antidepressants widely to children and teens, generalizing from the success of Prozac with adults to pediatric patients. (The first generation of antidepressants, the tricyclics like imipramine, weren't effective in children and weren't prescribed for them, even after child and teen depression was recognized in the mid-1970s, and diagnoses became much more common in the 1980s. The other early class of antidepressants, monoamine oxidase inhibitors or MAOIs, had potentially fatal side effects that made them a poor choice for treating children's depression.)

Bipolar disorder wasn't considered a possibility for kids until the 1990s, and so, in the absence of "manic-depressive" kids, you didn't have children taking bipolar medication. (As you would later, in vastly increasing numbers.) As far as ADHD drugs went—although the stimulant Benzedrine had been shown, as far back as the late 1930s, to work wonders for hyperactive kids with impulse control problems, and though Ritalin had been on the market since the 1970s, it wasn't really until the mid-1990s, when the understanding of ADHD expanded to include girls, teenagers, and inattentive children generally, that prescriptions of stimulants really skyrocketed.

These changes are popularly understood as reflecting the pharmaceutical industry's stupendous success in widening its markets in the 1990s, particularly once direct-to-consumer drug advertising was permitted at the end of the decade. There is undoubtedly some truth to that idea. But it's not the whole story.

The fact is, from the 1980s onwards, child psychiatrists were able to offer parents more treatments that worked. There were an expanding array of stimulants (and, eventually, nonstimulants) for ADHD, new antidepressants for depression, anxiety, and obsessive-compulsive disorder, and also cognitive behavioral therapy, which over the decades would prove to bring meaningful change to children with depression and anxiety disorders.

Doctors were also, in the "age of the brain," able to give parents a reprieve. They could explain that children with mental health issues were suffering from biological disorders, not bad parenting. As doctors' focus of treatment shifted from unraveling familial conflict—conscious and unconscious—to addressing symptoms and changing behavior, parents could be drawn in more easily and productively as partners. And they were.

Is it so surprising, then, that "suddenly" there were all these kids with mental health issues?

Doctors were able to see them. Parents were willing to see them. Schools and society were seeing them. All of a sudden, kids with "issues" were highly visible. The world, for better or for worse, had woken up to their existence.

The notion of visibility—who was seen and how they were seen—is, I believe, the key to understanding why it appears that there were virtually no kids with mental health issues in the past, and why it seems that they're all over today. There's a much greater awareness of the existence of mental illness in children now. There are more ways to diagnose and treat kids. (The two go hand in hand. As the medical historian Edward Shorter has written: "Physicians prefer to diagnose conditions they can treat rather than those they can't.") There's still stigma, but the abject shame of having a mentally ill child has greatly lessened. And there are vastly fewer kids in mental hospitals now than there were in the postwar past: In more recent decades the average pediatric stay on a psych ward declined from more than forty days in 1988, to about ten days in 2001.

Kids with serious problems are no longer routinely institutionalized because, as is the case with adults, they're kept functioning with medication. Kids with mental health issues are in school—in much greater numbers now than in the past. As late as 1975, when the Education for All Handicapped Children Act—a precursor to today's Individuals with Disabilities Education Act—was first enacted, many states barred from school children with disabilities, including emotionally disturbed or "mentally retarded" kids (a catchall appellation that included many children who today would be considered autistic).

"Almost a million children with disabilities received no education at all, and only seventeen states provided an education to even half of the known physically or mentally disabled children," historian Steven Mintz notes, in *Huck's Raft: A History of American Childhood.* "Until the mid 1970s most states allowed school districts to refuse to enroll students they considered 'ineducable.'"

Unable to attend public school, severely learning-disabled or autistic children in the past became invisible. Now, they are seen. Now, thanks to medication, children with emotional, behavioral, and developmental disorders go to places like sleepaway camp and college. They live broader, richer lives. Some might say more challenging lives. More visible lives, certainly.

The story isn't normally told this way. The news is never framed as: "Kids Who Would Have Stayed Home Now Given Fuller Access to Childhood." It's instead given sure-to-be-most-e-mailed headlines like "Checklist for Camp: Bug Spray. Sunscreen. Pills." Or, more bluntly: "Young Minds Under Attack."

The framing is incredibly important. Because it provides the context to the story of kids' mental health in our time that preconditions the story's meaning. It determines what we see when we look at the kids being diagnosed with and treated for mental disorders. And what we see, of course, is what we believe.

The question now—the question that reflects greatly back upon us as a society—is what we do with that vision.

· 3 ·

An Epidemic of Supposition

"I regard it as a public health crisis.
It's an epidemic, if you will."

MARTHA HELLANDER, THEN-RESEARCH DIRECTOR FOR THE CHILD AND ADOLESCENT BIPOLAR FOUNDATION, ON AMERICAN RADIOWORKS' "A MIND OF THEIR OWN," APRIL 19, 2005

"Bipolar disorder is the flavor of the month
in the diagnosis of children."

DR. RACHEL KLEIN, A PROFESSOR OF CHILD AND ADOLESCENT PSYCHIATRY AT THE NEW YORK UNIVERSITY SCHOOL OF MEDICINE, LATER ON THE SAME SHOW

The autism "epidemic" provides a very good example of how a disorder's becoming visible can lead to the perception that it has become greatly more common. As anthropologist Roy Richard Grinker tells the story in his 2007 book, *Unstrange Minds: Remapping the World of Autism*, the very dramatic rise in autism diagnoses over the past generation—when the official prevalence of autism in children has hopped from one in 2,000 to 5,000 before the 1990s, to one in 150 to 500 today—can to a very large extent be explained by radical changes in the way the disorder has been seen.

Back in 1943, when child psychiatrist Leo Kanner first described autism as a condition combining severe social and language impairments with strange repetitive behaviors, the disorder was believed to be extremely rare, occurring in fewer than three in 10,000 children. Kanner's definition, though, was based on observations of very severely disabled patients, not the variously affected children who show the wide range of behaviors and social and language impairments that are classed together under the umbrella category of "autism spectrum disorders" today.

Kanner's autism diagnosis was, from the start, inconsistently applied and far from universally accepted by psychiatrists. Throughout the postwar years in America, kids with the symptoms we now consider typical of autism were given other diagnoses. Some were called schizophrenic or mentally retarded. Others were given labels like "non-specific developmental delay," "brain dysfunction," "obsessive-compulsive disorder with brain dysfunction," or "seizure disorder."

DSM-III in 1980 changed all that, creating an official name and a set of symptoms for autism. *DSM-III R*, a 1987 revision, changed the diagnostic criteria in such a way that about one-third more children came under the umbrella of what were by then being called autism spectrum disorders. Afterward, diagnoses started to climb. They really took off, however, in the early 1990s, when, for the first time, public schools began using autism as a reporting category to the federal government as part of their compliance with the Individuals with Disabilities Education Act, which guaranteed every child a free and "appropriate" education in the least restrictive environment.

Autism diagnoses then soared. From 1991 to 2006, there was a 3,500 percent increase in American children identified as autistic in special-education programs, noted autism specialist Paul T. Shattuck and epidemiologist Maureen Durkin in a *New York Times* op-ed in 2007. It was an explosion in diagnosing that looked like, and was often called, an "epidemic." But what it really was, Shattuck and Durkin argued, was a perfect example of "diagnostic substitution." In public school reporting, they wrote, "the increase in autism was completely offset by a decrease in the prevalence of children considered 'cognitively disabled' or 'learning disabled.'"

The recategorization of children was one reason behind the rapid and seemingly stratospheric rise in autism diagnoses. Another was that there was, after 1991, a new impetus to identify autistic children in order to secure them vital services as early as possible. "Older studies used narrow definitions of autism and were generally based on counting the number of patients in a clinic or hospital with diagnoses of autism," Shattuck and Durkin explained. "Modern methods use broader criteria and leave no stone unturned in the effort to find every autistic child in a defined geographical area, including those not previously given a diagnosis. This virtually guarantees that new estimates will be higher than previous ones, even if the underlying prevalence of the condition has not changed. It's hardly a surprise," they concluded, "that looking harder to find children with disabilities has resulted in more diagnoses."

The basic outlines of the autism story hold true for other mental disorders, like depression or ADHD or bipolar disorder, that in recent years have frequently been called "epidemic" by both believers and nonbelievers in the reality of the diagnoses. The same general rule—that you find what you look for (or don't find what you don't look for)—strongly applies.

There were no kids with Asperger's when there was no Asperger's diagnosis. (It entered the *DSM* for the first time in 1994. Before that, kids with the disorder's signature combination of normal or even high intelligence and major social deficits were just diagnosed—by their peers—as "weird.")

You didn't see any kids with depression when it was believed that children couldn't suffer from depression. Once that belief changed, the percentage of depressed children appeared to skyrocket—rising from about zero in the early 1970s to the 2 to 15 percent of kids (depending on who's counting) who are said to suffer from the disorder today. There weren't any bipolar kids until psychiatrists in the mid-1990s, influenced chiefly by the work of Harvard University's Joseph Biederman at Massachusetts General Hospital, began saying that there were. And suddenly (or not so suddenly, if your historical memory stretched back to Emil Kraepelin), up to 1 percent of children were said to suffer from the disorder.

When what is today called ADHD—and conceived of as a constellation of symptoms and behaviors grouped around inattention, problems with impulse control, poor working memory, issues of self-regulation, and other cognitive and social deficits—was simply thought of as hyperactivity, not all that many children suffered from the disorder. (In 1976, although Ritalin was already on the market, only between 1.5 and 2 percent of school-aged children were taking psychostimulants.) When epidemiological surveys later looked to track the number of kids with ADHD, but only counted the number with the "combined type" of the disorder (hyperactivity plus inattention), a still-modest 3 to 5 percent of children were said to be affected. When, more recently, epidemiologists started including kids with the uniquely "inattentive" subtype of ADHD (no hyperactivity—the kind of ADHD you typically see in girls and in teens), prevalence numbers nearly doubled, so that today, ADHD is believed to be present in about 8 percent of kids. Epidemiologists say that that increase is largely, if not entirely, a result of changed diagnostic patterns.

The inclusion of children with ADHD in the category of students eligible for special-education services under the Individuals with Disabilities Education Act (IDEA) also helped. Once again, simply put, it's a seek-and-ye-shall-find phenomenon.

Increased visibility, aided by more incentives to diagnose kids, and profound changes in how parents, teachers, and doctors look at and label kids who have problems are all key factors driving the widespread perception that kids today are suddenly showing up with all kinds of new and surprising "issues." But they are probably not the only factors, and "diagnostic substitution" is undoubtedly not the whole story.

Some experts believe that certain mental health disorders really are on the rise in children. Many say, for example, that depression really is increasing in kids as well as in adults. This belief is based in large part on a series of "cohort" studies from Yale University and the National Institute of Mental Health that in the mid-1980s found that successive generations of Americans born after World War II seemed to have both a greater incidence and earlier onset of depression. One study showed that people born around 1910 had only a 1.3 percent chance of having a major depressive episode, whereas those born after 1960 had a 5.3 percent chance, and there was an approximately tenfold increase in risk for depression in each successive generational group. Another study of families with depression showed higher rates of severe clinical depression in younger relatives than older ones.

Others say that anxiety really is increasing. Jean Twenge, a San Diego State University psychologist, most notably made this argument, in a chapter called "The Age of Anxiety (and Depression, and Loneliness)" in her 2006 book, *Generation Me: Why Today's Young Americans Are More Confident, Assertive, Entitled–and More Miserable Than Ever Before.* "The number of teens aged 14–16 who agreed that 'Life is a strain for me much of the time' quadrupled between the early 1950s and 1989," she wrote. "A 2001 poll found almost 75% of teenagers said they felt nervous or stressed at least some of the time, and half said they often felt this way. One out of three college freshmen reported feeling 'frequently overwhelmed' in 2001, twice as many as in the 1980s."

And others believe that bipolar disorder, diagnoses of which skyrocketed in kids over the past fifteen years, is truly increasing in children as well. The chief popularizer of this view is Demitri Papolos, an associate professor of psychiatry at the Albert Einstein College of Medicine in New York City, who used data from the Yale cohort studies to argue, in his 2002 book, *The Bipolar Child,* that bipolar disorder is increasing and coming on much earlier in children now than it did in prior generations.

There are lots of theories to back up these assertions. Some emphasize psychosocial factors: life is more depressing than ever before. Life is more anxious-making. Life is more distracting—and all these factors make living today much harder for kids with a genetic tendency toward mental health issues. Some stress genetics—particularly the concept of genetic anticipation, which holds that mental disorders come on earlier and with more severity when they're passed down through the generations.

One iteration of the genetic anticipation concept that I've always found particularly intriguing is the notion of "assortative mating"—like marrying like—a practice that has vastly increased in recent decades, as people have come to marry mates they meet in college, at work, and through shared interests, thus linking up, to a formerly unprecedented degree, with similarly minded (and neurologically wired) life partners.

Demitri Papolos, for one, believes that assortative mating could well explain, to some extent at least, why we're seeing many more diagnoses of bipolar disorder in kids.

"Assortative mating," he told me, "has increased with the mobilization of society since the interstate highways were built in the fifties and the use of air flight which has contributed to the breakdown of local kinship structures. In the past," Papolos said, "spouse selection took into consideration knowledge of the partner's family. If Aunt Emma went around the bend, or Uncle Albert had been institutionalized, you might think twice if psychiatric illness also ran in your family. Now, few couples have much of a clue as to the medical and psychiatric history of families they are marrying into and frequently [in the case of bipolar disorder, 35 percent] individuals marry others of similar temperament and background. In our studies, age of onset before the age of ten is invariably associated with bilineal transmission."

Another proponent of the "assortative mating" theory is Simon Baron-Cohen, the director of the Autism Research Centre at the University of Cambridge (and a cousin of *Borat* and *Brüno* star Sacha Baron Cohen) who believes it could be one explanation for what he has called "the mystery" of autism in our time. His research has found that disproportionate numbers of autistic children have grandfathers, on both their maternal and paternal sides, who were engineers, and economists. The children's parents—mothers and fathers both—also tend to have minds that show strong "systemizing" tendencies of the kind you generally see in economists, engineers, and mathematicians. They also, he has found, tend to score above average on questionnaires that measure autistic traits. The obsessions of autism, then, he believes, could be seen as an overload of such genetic tendencies—"very intense systemizing at work."

Explaining further, he wrote me in a 2006 e-mail, "The key concept is 'assortative mating' of strong systemizers, meaning . . . that systemizers are attracted to one another and are nowadays finding and meeting one another and having families, more often."

Assortative mating is a fascinating concept, one that's been taken up by a wide range of social scientists in different contexts. Some evolutionary psychologists have warned that the pumping-up of certain kids' genes through the now common practice of high-level professionals marrying other high-level professionals will increase our country's class-related achievement gap. Eating-disorder experts have wondered whether the new trends in spousal selection of the past thirty-odd years can partly explain the increased and earlier incidence of anorexia nervosa in today's girls. (Too many perfectionists marrying perfectionists, too little "hybrid vigor.")

After talking to Madeline Levine, a psychologist in wealthy Marin County, and the Columbia University psychologist Suniya Luthar, both of whom have written of a seeming "epidemic" of mental health issues among today's most privileged youth, I came to wonder whether assortative mating was playing a role in that population as well. Levine notes in her 2006 book, *The Price of Privilege,* that well-off teens today are greatly outpacing their middle-class peers in rates of cigarette smoking, depression, alcohol and drug abuse, anxiety, rule-breaking, and psychosomatic disorders, like headaches and stomach problems. Thirty to 40 percent of twelve- to eighteen-year-olds from affluent homes show such "troubling psychological symptoms," she says. As many as 22 percent of adolescent girls from these well-off families—three times the national rate—suffer from clinical depression, and by the end of high school, fully one-third of these girls exhibit clinically significant signs of anxiety.

Levine and Luthar (whose research informed much of *The Price of Privilege*) indict upper-middle-class cultural values, pressures, stresses, and parenting practices in particular as causes for all this unexpectedly common mental pathology. But I wonder if genetics don't factor in, too.

In no other generation, after all, have doctors, lawyers, bankers—the high achievers generally who fill our nation's upper middle class—married their professional peers, as the current group of affluent parents has done. And, thanks to this assortative mating, no other generational subgroup of kids has gotten such a double whammy of the traits that brought their parents their success. Some of these traits are positive, like intelligence. But some are not. Some things that drive success—like anxiety, mania, and an obsessive singularity of vision—can be mental demons.

Of course, that is just supposition.

But supposition is all we really have in trying to answer the big question that so often pops up in discussions of kids with issues: Are there really more of them today, or are we merely seeing and counting them differently?

The unfortunate truth is: Hard data just doesn't exist. The research that could provide solid answers—epidemiological studies conducted in a parallel manner over time, asking the same questions, looking for the same disorders, using consistent language and definitions—for the most part doesn't exist. The precise survey questions that are asked today about kids weren't asked in the past, which makes the issue of whether and to what extent children suffered from mental illness a tree-falling-in-the-forest kind of a question: If nobody counted them, were they there? (As Gabrielle Carlson, a professor of child and adolescent psychiatry at Stony Brook University School of Medicine, once pointed out, "Not asking is not the same as not having.")

And for every researcher who believes there has been a real increase in a certain mental disorder, there is another one saying that, in fact, there hasn't. Take the question of depression, for example: There are some epidemiological studies looking for depression in children going back to the mid-1970s. In 2006, the Duke University epidemiologist E. Jane Costello reviewed studies of close to 60,000 children and adults who were born between 1965 and 1996 and had at some point in their lives undergone at least one structured diagnostic psychiatric interview. She found no sign of any real increase in depression in kids over the past thirty years.

Costello suggested that there were problems with the "cohort" studies that are so often cited to back claims that depression is on the rise. For one thing, she said, they relied on people's recollections of how they had felt long before, rather than on research data gathered contemporaneously. This was perhaps not very reliable, she wrote, as people tend to sugarcoat their early memories, and also, simply, to forget how they felt. As for clinician observations that more depressed children were coming into their offices than ever before: Costello offered that perhaps in an era when depression among people of all ages is better recognized and less stigmatized, more parents were bringing more children in for treatment.

"Thirty years of research suggests that, for as far back as we have reliable assessments, a similar proportion of children have been depressed, albeit largely unrecognized by clinicians," she concluded. "If more depressed children are being identified, or are receiving antidepressant medication, this is more likely to be the result of increased sensitivity to a long-standing problem than of an 'epidemic.'"

In 2007, another team of doctors writing in *The Journal of the American Medical Association* threw their weight behind this conclusion. "No clear evidence documents a secular increase in prevalence of depression in children and youth, although greater numbers in recent years have been identified and receive services," they wrote.

There is similar disagreement on the question of anxiety. A number of the clinicians I spoke with said they were seeing many more anxious children than ever before in their office practices. But it wasn't clear what those observations meant. More anxious kids than ever before? Or more parents recognizing the signs of anxiety and feeling that their children needed help? And who's to say that our indisputably anxious times are actually *more* anxious than other periods in history? The Great Depression was horribly anxious-making. As was World War II. As were polio or influenza outbreaks. The list could go on and on. In the past, however, no one was conducting telephone surveys to see if the nation's children were cracking up under duress.

"In 1850, kids were anxious," Harvard psychologist Jerome Kagan once told me, speaking from the perspective of more than a half-century spent teaching and practicing child psychology. "But they were anxious about other things."

There's plenty of research to indicate that, in many ways, despite the problems of elite kids, children and teens are, overall, actually doing *better* than they did in the past. Teen pregnancy, school violence, and crime have all been on the decline for decades, as are cigarette smoking and illegal drug and alcohol use. The teen suicide rate fell 30 percent from 1990 to 2003, to levels not seen since the 1970s. (It started rising again in 2004, after the FDA issued a "black box" warning that antidepressants like Prozac and Paxil could put children and teens at greater risk of suicidal thoughts and behavior, and doctors sharply curtailed their prescribing of these and other SSRIs.)

Teenagers today miss fewer days of school and are more likely to graduate from high school and college than were the baby boomers. The percentage of college freshmen who find themselves "frequently depressed" fell from a high of 11 percent in 1988 to just 7 percent in 2005 and 2006. Higher percentages of high school seniors now say they are "'very happy,' are having fun, enjoy the fast pace of modern life, view the future optimistically and feel it's important to make a contribution to society" than did their predecessors in the 1970s, Mike Males, a sociologist, reviewing these numbers, reported in the *Los Angeles Times* in 2007. Fewer, he wrote, say they feel "lonely, left out and 'no good at all.'"

How to make sense of all these apples and oranges—these varying indicators of distress or well-being that can be shuffled and assembled to tell virtually any story you want? Perhaps only by realizing that they are, indeed, elements of story, and that the narratives we weave them into have at least as much to say about how we feel about childhood in our anxious and depressing times as they do about today's children and teens.

The debate over whether there are, in fact, more bipolar children now or whether large numbers of children are just being inappropriately diagnosed with the disorder and medicated has a different kind of urgency; in fact, it's perhaps the most hotly contested issue in child psychiatry today. And that's because there has been such a sudden, enormous, and, many say, scientifically ungrounded rise in the number of bipolar diagnoses, and because the medications used to treat bipolar disorder in kids—anticonvulsants, which also work as mood stabilizers, and second-generation or "atypical" antipsychotics—are so powerful and new and potentially dangerous.

As I noted earlier, up until about fifteen years ago, most psychiatrists believed that bipolar disorder didn't exist in kids before the late teen years. Then, after doctors at Massachusetts General Hospital started finding it in children as young as age two, diagnoses exploded, increasing a massive fortyfold from 1994 to 2003. By 2007, half a million to a million American children were said to suffer from the disorder. By 2008, approximately one-fourth of all pediatric patients discharged from hospitals with psychiatric diagnoses were leaving with a bipolar label.

Discussions of this issue tend to be heavily clouded by the fact that this increase occurred at the same time that the new generation of "atypical" antipsychotics came on the market—a conjunction of events complicated further by the fact that some of the doctors who most visibly promoted the meds as an off-label way to treat emotionally volatile kids turned out to be in the pay of drugmakers. The latter issue is a scandal—to which I'll return later—but it's also really just one part of a much more complicated story. There are—there have always been—a certain number of kids with wild mood swings and out-of-control behavior whose destructiveness and disruptiveness drive their parents to despair. Twenty-five years ago, these children were diagnosed with conduct disorders. Before that, if they were brought in for treatment and not just sent to reform schools, they would perhaps have been called schizophrenic. In either case, they would have been hospitalized for weeks or months or years, depending on the decade, and they would have been given powerful antipsychotic drugs like Haldol or Thorazine. If they became violent and committed crimes, they would have been jailed.

Today, except in the most extreme cases, if children like these are hospitalized at all, it's very briefly. They live at home—and are given powerful antipsychotics like Risperdal and Zyprexa. That these kids are very sick is not—among the mental health specialists who work with them, at least—in question.

"These kids do have serious problems. It's not as though the kids who are being labeled as bipolar aren't ill," Mark Olfson, the Columbia University psychiatrist who discovered the fortyfold increase in bipolar diagnoses, told me.

But are they—as they have come so often to be labeled—bipolar?

Many experts are skeptical. There's something fishy, some point out, about the fact that, while mood disorders occur predominantly in women, most of the new juvenile bipolar diagnoses being made today are of boys. (Adult diagnoses now are two-thirds female; child diagnoses of bipolar are two-thirds male.)

It isn't right, some argue, that to fit kids into the bipolar diagnosis, clinicians in practice often fiddle with the criteria for diagnosis—"a somewhat tautological undertaking," in the words of Jennifer Harris, a clinical instructor at Harvard Medical School. The significant changes in mood that are the signature feature of bipolar disorder, for example, are said to commonly take place over a matter of hours for bipolar kids, while in adults cycles usually last a period of weeks or months. "Mania" is said by some juvenile bipolar advocates to look very different in kids than it does in adults: to come across as irritability, rather than a greatly elevated mood, and the landmark adult symptom of "grandiosity" can simply take the form of a child's thinking he or she knows better than adults.

Skeptics also point out that the patients being diagnosed as kids should turn out to be bipolar as adults. Yet research has shown that extreme, persistent irritability—the symptom that often leads doctors to diagnose children and teens as bipolar—is not a valid predictor of later bipolar disorder. What irritability does correlate with, later on, is an increased risk of anxiety and depression. Which has led some experts to wonder whether many of the out-of-control, volatile kids who today get the bipolar diagnosis (and meds) aren't in fact exhibiting a juvenile form of depression in the first place.

This theory was given weight in 2001 by a study, conducted in a private psychiatric hospital in Westchester County, New York, where researchers carefully reinterviewed children who'd come in with bipolar diagnoses from doctors in their communities. They found that fully half of those "bipolar" kids weren't bipolar at all. They were depressed—severely depressed.

Ellen Leibenluft, chief of the section on Bipolar Spectrum Disorders in the Mood and Anxiety Disorders Program at the National Institute of Mental Health, has seen this over and over again. Since 2003 she has been closely following a group of one hundred kids whose chronic irritability, negative mood, and frequent, violent temper outbursts would normally, these days, get them diagnosed as bipolar. In fact, about 60 percent of the kids were diagnosed as bipolar out in their communities—falsely, Leibenluft believes.

"Bipolar disorder is very rare in children," she told me, "but there's a much larger group that struggles with very extreme irritability, flying off the handle, having great difficulty regulating their mood on a day-to-day basis, and very extreme behavior."

Leibenluft has suggested a new diagnosis for these children. She calls it "severe mood dysregulation." Her work and other research have indicated that a lot of the kids who fit the severe mood dysregulation category grow up to be severely depressed. Childhood is for many of them a time of sheer agony. "These kids are really hurting and are every bit as sick as the bipolar kids, whatever we call them," she said.

What these kids are called—how they are seen—is of vital importance. Because it determines the kind of treatment they're given. Using anticonvulsants and "atypical" antipsychotics, which can have dangerous side effects like big weight gains and metabolic changes, can be dangerously inappropriate, or, at the very least, inadequate for them: The Westchester County study found that the falsely diagnosed bipolar kids who'd been prescribed, and continued to take, anticonvulsants got noticeably worse over time.

Leibenluft noted that getting away from the bipolar diagnosis opens up avenues for treatment—psychopharmacological and not—that may offer real hope without the known dangers of atypical antipsychotic use. "Based on the kids we see, I think most of them would still need medications," she told me. But, she added, "You are looking at a different category of meds if you're looking at anxiety and depression rather than bipolar disorder, and you get into the whole category of nonpharmacological interventions. Could you train kids to attend away from what's upsetting them to something else? In anxiety, they could attend away from what's making them anxious. In depression, there's cognitive behavioral therapy to learn how you reframe what's going on so it's not so depressing or frustrating."

It seems to me that, as a society, we would do well to start learning to reframe how we think about what's going on with the kids being diagnosed with issues like bipolar disorder, too. Too much mental energy now is going into debating whether or not these "new" children's disorders are real. Not enough is going into finding ways to help children who are visibly suffering do better.

This could, in so many ways, be a moment rich in promise. As a report from the National Institute of Mental Health stated nearly a decade ago, "Years ago, people with mental illness were doomed to live without prospect for active and productive lives." Now, the authors concluded, "scientific advances" can "offer hope." Yet very few people feel hopeful right now, scanning the landscape of children with mental health issues.

Outside observers see an incomprehensible "epidemic"; parents of children with mental illness see stigma, confusion, and roadblocks to care. We truly are in the throes of a "brave new world" kind of a moment, using the phrase as it's defined by *The American Heritage Dictionary*, to mean "A world or realm of radically transformed existence, especially one in which technological progress has both positive and negative results." This is a time when scientific advances have outpaced our abilities to use them well. It's a time when there's a general sense of wool being pulled over people's eyes, and a feeling, almost, of conspiracy: that something is being done to kids (and adults) by occult forces seeking to pathologize, drug, and control them. The fears contained in those beliefs are worsened by talk of "epidemics"—either by boosters seeking to raise awareness and funds for the particular illnesses that occupy or obsess them, or by social critics trying to build a case for the general corruption and misery of youth today.

Overall, it adds up to a lot of suspicion and doubt and skepticism and a poisonous level of parent blame that has far outlasted the prior prejudices of mental health professionals. Nowhere is this more dramatically true than on the question of psychotropic medication.

· 4 ·

Aren't They All *on Medication?*

"There can be no argument that we are in the midst of a legal-drugging epidemic."

ARIANNA HUFFINGTON, APRIL 2, 2007

In March 2007, a few months after the scales-falling-from-my-eyes moment in the coffeehouse, I wrote about my profound change of heart online for *The New York Times*.

"What if children's troublesome symptoms are *not* their truest form of self-expression?" I asked, in a column called "Second Thoughts."

"What if, in the past, it really wasn't so great to leave 'quirky' kids to tough it out on their own? What if recycling a watered-down version of sixties-era radical thinking about psychiatry and the normalizing evils of mainstream society isn't the best approach to take in today's world? What if the whole topic deserves a new kind of radical rethinking?"

The response from readers was much as you might expect. Parents of children with issues, and adults who as kids had suffered from what we would today call issues, were, by and large, thrilled.

Other people were not.

"It's too bad you didn't continue on to write that first book, Judith. You could have exposed one of the greatest frauds in a generation," wrote one reader. Others talked about "unaware capitalism," the need for organic food, the toxicity of TV, the perils of working motherhood, and the general sickness of our performance-mad culture.

"There is no doubt in my mind that the upper class today is freaking out its children by their obsessive focus on status and a very narrow definition of achievement, and also that many parents simply do not have the will to act as grown-ups and deny their children anything," was a typical comment.

One of the people who wrote to the *Times* was Mindy Lewis, the writer and artist I mentioned earlier who, as a rebellious teenager in 1967, had been diagnosed with schizophrenia, then institutionalized and treated with Thorazine for more than two years.

We spoke by phone in the spring of 2008. She told me her story—how she'd been anxious and unhappy, how her mother, signing away her parental authority when she handed her daughter over to psychiatrists, had been overwhelmed and scared. She warned against the dangers of trusting mental health professionals and railed against the practice of medicating kids.

I interrupted her. I wanted to be sure she understood my perspective. I didn't want her to spend hours talking to me only to later open my book and feel betrayed.

I told her that, while I sympathized with her story deeply, I didn't necessarily think that what she'd lived through was analogous to what most kids receiving psychiatric care were experiencing today. I said I thought that child psychiatry had evolved. I thought doctors had learned lessons from the errors of past generations. I thought—based on the research I had done since writing "Second Thoughts"—that most of the kids taking medication today benefitted from it, and that the whole story of "drugging kids" was being overblown.

There was a moment of silence.

But weren't *they all* on medication? she asked bewilderedly.

It's not an uncommon belief.

You hear it said all the time of kids today: "They're *all* on medication."

The "all" is a conversation-starter. It creates a connection that feels noble: You are united in a common cause against all those crazy parents and doctors out there who are handing out meds like candy.

I used to have a lot of these sorts of conversations. But once I had my change of heart, the interactions altered.

"Who, exactly?" I would say, if, for example, a mom told me that "all" the boys in her son's school were, of course, on meds. "How many do you know of, personally?"

The conversation would end. There would be a chill. I never got any answers, once I started asking for an accounting of who "all" was actually on medication. Usually, the parent couldn't count off a single child.

It's very easy to believe that kids today are "all" on drugs when you look at the dizzying array of damning numbers that have been making headlines over the past ten years.

A sampling:

> ***"Prescriptions for Ritalin have increased 600 percent."***
>
> *"Our Children Suffer When We Try to Medicate Their Troubles Away,"* Fort Wayne News-Sentinel

> ***"By fifth grade, 18 to 20 percent of white boys were receiving ADHD medication."***
>
> *"Pills or Patience: More Children Are Being Given Drugs for Behavioral and Emotional Problems,"* The Sacramento Bee

> *"Between the early '90s and 2001, the prescription rate of antidepressants for those under 18 more than tripled."*
>
> "*The Antidepressant Dilemma,*"
> The New York Times Magazine

> *"A study released this summer showed a more than fivefold increase in the number of antipsychotic drugs prescribed to youth."*
>
> "*Don't Crush Budding Einsteins,*"
> The Fresno Bee

> *"From 1987 through 1996, psychotropic drug use among children and teens nearly tripled."*
>
> "*Young and Alone,*"
> Los Angeles Times

The problem is, however, the numbers don't really tell much of a story. Some—like the often alleged 600 percent increase in Ritalin use in the 1990s, and the frequently reported "fact" that up to a fifth of fifth-grade white boys are on ADHD meds—have turned out, upon examination, to be just plain wrong.

Others—as was the case with the increases in diagnoses I discussed in the last chapter—simply lack meaning, or lend themselves to easily distorted meanings, unless you put them into context. Taking a few examples from the news:

How meaningful is it to know that, in the 1990s, antidepressant use tripled, if you don't know that prior to the 1990s—i.e., before the age of Prozac—antidepressants were pretty much never given to kids at all? (The first-generation drugs had serious side effects, were fatal in overdose, and did not prove in children to be more effective than placebo.) How huge does that tripling seem if you find out that, at the end of this nothing-to-something transition, there was still only a tiny percentage of kids—I've seen numbers ranging from one-half of a percent to 1.3 percent—taking antidepressant medication? And that this percentage on meds—up to 1 or 2 percent today—is far smaller than the 2 percent or 8 percent or 15 percent (depending on who's counting) who are said to suffer from depression?

How meaningful is it to know, as has been widely reported, that up to 25 percent of foster children in some states are taking psychotropic medication, if you don't also consider the flip side: other data showing that, within this same population of kids, serious mental health issues are rampant—and usually go untreated?

In 2007, an Associated Press story on the phenomenon of over-medicating foster kids circulated widely, with one child-welfare advocate quoted as saying that meds were a "chemical sledgehammer that makes children easier to manage." But what didn't get around much was the fact that as many as 60 percent of foster kids suffer from mental illness. And less than half of the foster children who show signs of serious mental disturbances ever receive medication.

These are often children who have been put through hell: abuse, neglect, domestic violence, abrupt separation, and loss. Often enough they have parents who themselves struggle with mental health issues or self-medicate against those issues with drugs or alcohol. In some cases—in one in four cases in the state of Virginia, a 2004 study found—it's *because* a child has mental health issues that he or she ends up in foster care in the first place.

While it is highly worrisome to know that too many now get medication—multiple medications—without therapy and without support for the traumas they've endured, it is more troubling to think of what happens to those who, like the vast majority of disadvantaged children, get no treatment at all. "You don't get a 'label,'" University of Michigan School of Public Health psychiatrist Don Vereen, who, while deputy director of the office of National Drug Control Policy in the Clinton administration saw psychotropic prescriptions for well-off children sharply rise while poorer children with mental health issues languished, undiagnosed, once told me. "But you'll end up in the criminal justice system." In fact, surveys have shown that about two-thirds of the inmates in our country's juvenile correction system have at least one mental illness.

I don't mean to minimize the seriousness of treating children with drugs that can increase suicidal thoughts (in the case of SSRIs), or are largely untested and known to have gravely serious side effects (as is true, for example, of atypical antipsychotics). I don't mean to be lending support to the practice of delivering psychotropic medication first to abused, neglected, or otherwise traumatized children and providing therapy later, if at all. I do not think children should be given medication lightly. In an ideal world, I would hope that none would receive medication without some additional kind of appropriate therapy or support.

In short, I do not mean to be providing an apologia for the drug companies or for physician practices or health plans that promote prescribing medication in a void, without comprehensive care. But I do want to draw attention to the intellectual void in which the arguments for the "legal-drugging" epidemic have been made. The numbers have, until now, done all the talking. And where there should have been context, there has been silence.

The silence is curious. Particularly when you consider how very loud the hysteria has been.

The basic arguments I have made here about antidepressants and about foster kids hold up generally for the whole issue of pediatric psychotropic drug use: The total number of kids taking these drugs is far smaller than most people think. And, even after decades of rapid increases, the percentage of kids taking meds is still just a fraction of the number of kids with psychiatric issues.

It comes down to this: Five percent of kids in America take psychotropic drugs.

Five to 20 percent have psychiatric issues.*

That, according to my math, just doesn't add up to a pattern of gross overmedication. The number of kids taking psychotropic medication has been greatly exaggerated in the public mind. Vastly overblown, too, have been assertions, replayed endlessly by critics in the echo chamber of the media, that kids with nothing wrong with them are being diagnosed and "drugged."

Some variation of this idea has been repeated so many times that it has become received wisdom: Fully 86 percent of Americans, a recent survey found, now believe that physicians are overmedicating children for nothing more than common behavior problems. But there's no evidence to show that this is more than very episodically true.

In 2006, the American Psychological Association—no particular friend to biological psychiatry—convened a special task force to take up the issue of overmedication. The psychologists soon found that doctors were too quick to medicate and tended too often to rely on medication without therapy in treating kids. But, said Dr. Ronald Brown, a professor of public health, psychology, and pediatrics at Temple University who headed up that task force, the committee also discovered that it wasn't true that kids with nothing wrong with them were being medicated. Perfectly healthy kids weren't being pathologized. Those being given meds really did have serious issues. "The literature is showing that basically the diagnoses are correct," he told me. "When you do surveillance, it's not overdiagnosis you see; if anything, it's underdiagnosis. Most kids don't get services. Access is poor and there's a lack of providers."

Two decades of survey research into ADHD diagnosing and stimulant use have led to a similar conclusion. *Some* overdiagnosis and overuse of medication do exist; one of the latest studies on the question found that

---

* The 5 percent being those with "extreme functional impairment," according to U.S. government statistics, the 20 percent being those with "at least minimum impairment."

3.3 percent of children who were taking meds shouldn't have been because researchers judged that they didn't really have the disorder. Yet, underdiagnosis and underuse of medication consistently show up in research as much bigger problems. Studies routinely find that only about half of kids with ADHD get any treatment for it at all, and that girls, minority children, and children with less-educated parents are less frequently treated still.

And while there is, and has long been, a big and problematic amount of geographical variation in the number of kids being diagnosed with ADHD (from a low of 5 percent in Colorado to high of 11.1 percent in Alabama at last count), the really huge numbers indicating gross overdiagnosis have never proven to be valid. When tested by research, the idea that a whole lot of kids are getting false ADHD diagnoses and consequent drug treatment hasn't held up.

The same holds true for antidepressants: There is some overuse, or inappropriate use in very young or very mildly affected kids. And there is much more underuse in, and underdiagnosis among, severely depressed kids. Indeed, depression is "among the least likely of all childhood mental health problems to receive treatment," a team of physicians and social scientists studying children's mental health services and social stigma concluded in 2007, noting that, because depressed children are generally not disruptive, their problems tend to be overlooked.

When it comes to atypical antipsychotics, there are real causes for alarm. Use of the drugs, most of which have not been approved for children and can cause serious metabolic changes and weight gain, increased fivefold from the mid-1990s to the mid-2000s. By 2003 just over half a million kids were taking the drugs, which are generally used to treat bipolar disorder and agitation and aggression in autistic kids. Half a million to a million kids had been diagnosed as bipolar—a trend that a great many psychiatrists regarded with skepticism. And yet, even the psychiatrists who have been the most active in investigating that rapid increase don't tend to believe that children with *nothing wrong with them* are being drugged up with these powerful meds.

Columbia University psychiatrist Mark Olfson, who established the recent fortyfold increase in bipolar diagnoses in children, has frequently spoken out to share his view that the diagnosing of bipolar disorder in kids has gotten out of hand. And yet, as I mentioned in the last chapter, he doesn't think that perfectly healthy kids are being labeled as bipolar. And he doesn't think that bipolar drugs are being handed out lightly, or completely inappropriately. "The drugs probably do help or else the kids wouldn't be treated in this way," he told me. "I don't fall into the camp of people who believe it's a grand conspiracy of drug companies and psychiatrists and parents. There are real risks of not treating these kids. The people who say they should just tough it out—I don't think that's a compassionate response. What's missing is the severity and amount of problems and the amount of pain. Parents are at their wits' end."

"The kids I'm treating are tortured by their symptoms," New York University Child Study Center director Harold Koplewicz, who harbors a great deal of doubt about the real prevalence of bipolar disorder in young children, said of the kids referred to him with a bipolar diagnosis. "You medicate symptoms to get them through it," he told me.

The fact of the matter is a large number of children are really suffering. Suffering so much that many are willing—and their parents are willing—to submit to the uncertainties and dangers of psychotropic medication. Why this basic fact, the reality of the pain that drives the decision to medicate, has so consistently been obscured from public view in the endless coverage there's been of the kids-and-meds issue is somewhat mysterious to me.

But then, maybe, once again, you just have to have the eyes to see it.

In early 2008, just as I was getting ready to write this book, I went to lunch with a reporter who covers the pharmaceutical industry. I was very familiar with his reporting; I'd been reading his stories for years. His coverage of the industry was exhaustive, damning, and, it seemed to me, impeccable.

I knew that we'd have some points to debate when we went to lunch. I knew he was highly skeptical about the reality of ADHD. I knew he thought the absolute worst of the pharmaceutical industry, and that he doubted that many of the psychotropic drugs on the market actually worked.

What I didn't realize was that we'd end up all but shouting at each other for close to two hours. He assailed me with questions:

How could I defend giving kids meds that weren't approved for their use and had terrible, sometimes deadly side effects?

How could I believe that any sorts of problems could ever justify their use?

How could I possibly believe that kids really had ADHD or depression in anywhere near the numbers indicated by the numbers of prescriptions written for stimulants and antidepressants?

How could I believe parents when they said they "had no choice" but to give their kids meds?

I shot back:

How could he believe parents would give their kids potentially very dangerous chemicals if they didn't have a damn good reason?

Why would they continue—why would they let their kids' doctors continue—to give them meds if the drugs didn't work?

Why was he so quick to assume that psychiatrists were charlatans?

And why did he have such an incredibly low opinion of parents?

This reporter had talked to a lot of parents. And what he saw, he said, were mothers who gave up on their children without trying. Who seemed motivated to medicate by exhaustion and embarrassment. "It was always an incident in a supermarket," he said, "with 'everyone staring' that pushed them over the edge. And when I was in their houses, the minute they thought there might be trouble, you know what they did? They closed the front door. They just didn't want the neighbors to hear."

He'd told me of moms who'd bragged to him how bipolar meds had raised their kids' grades from Bs to As. And of dads who rolled their eyes, telling him—the minute the moms' backs were turned—that if it were up to them, their kids wouldn't be taking medication at all. Because it was all "bullshit."

Where did you find these parents? I asked.

He referred me to the Internet.

But that wasn't what I meant.

I knew where to find parents of kids with mental health issues. Once I'd started asking around for people to interview, I'd had more offers than I could handle.

What I meant was: Where did you find parents who used antipsychotics or mood stabilizers to raise their kids' grades? Where did you find ones who turned eagerly to drugs to curb what were, essentially, temper tantrums? How did you find ones who actually *wanted* to give their kids medication?

The parents I'd talked to—and I'd talked to many dozens by that point—didn't fit that description at all. They'd come to accept psychiatric diagnoses of their kids brokenheartedly. The decision to medicate their kids was almost always one of the hardest they'd ever made in their lives, and they'd come to it only when they felt they had exhausted all other options. I never encountered anyone who medicated his or her child for trivial reasons of convenience or higher achievement. I never found anyone who received a child's bad report card, hopped on the Internet, and stormed into a doctor's office demanding a prescription. More typically, it was a child's pain, not his performance shortfalls, that caught a parent's attention.

Some parents *did* speak to me proudly of better grades once their kids were on medication, but with the exception of one girl with ADHD (whose prior B grades had been accompanied by an hour of crying and screaming every night), the improvements consisted generally of a change from failing to not failing.

Sometimes kids did start to get As once they were on medication. For the parents this was like an unexpected little miracle, the icing on the cake. And it was so much easier to talk about things like good grades than to dredge up all the terrible, painful memories of times past, relive all the guilt about wrong turns or missed opportunities, all the fear, then the hope, then the chastened acceptance of a child's challenges and limitations.

People don't generally open up about these kinds of things. The subject is a Pandora's box, emotionally. You want to be absolutely sure of your audience before you start. Like the moms closing the doors of their homes when their children started to spiral out of control, the parents I spoke with had witnessed things they didn't easily want to offer up to an outsider's scrutiny. They knew perfectly well how their parenting decisions were perceived by the public at large; the last thing they needed was to open themselves up to more criticism and condemnation. When I decided to tell their story—as opposed to dictating it based on my prejudices and preconceptions—I knew I had to approach them very carefully.

I wrote first to the parents I hoped to interview, and shared with them the journey I'd made in coming to have "second thoughts" about my beliefs on children's mental health issues. The parents related to my story. Most had made the same journey themselves.

"I went into this with so much fear and so many moral misgivings," the mother of an eleven-year-old boy with the inattentive type of ADHD in Los Angeles told me about the beginning of her quest to figure out why her intellectually gifted son couldn't function in school. He couldn't focus in class, couldn't finish his work, was "spacey" and immature, and had a tendency to miss social cues. His pediatrician worried he was headed for life as "the weird kid." When he began falling below grade-level standards on some standardized tests, his third-grade teacher said she was "extremely alarmed."

"My knee-jerk reaction was: it's not my son, it's you," the mom said.

"It was a school where they give homework in kindergarten. There was a lot of craft stuff, but it was very regimented. There was this need to fit a standard. The principal even told me once: 'Kids who are outside of the box are getting shortchanged. No Child Left Behind is leaving a lot of kids behind because teachers have to stick to the curriculum.'"

Sure that her son was a square peg in a round hole, the mother put off having him tested. And then, after he'd been tested and was diagnosed with ADHD, she resisted giving him medication. Why, she thought, should she change him to fit an unworthy system?

"I was sort of convinced it was like *One Flew Over the Cuckoo's Nest*, where the problem was as much the system as the individual in the system, and in the end the system fucked him over," she said. "I just have that inherent vision in my system."

I heard this kind of distrust and disbelief—this sense that, in an "off-kilter" world, as the L.A. mother put it, you can hardly expect a child to thrive—over and over again.

A Washington, D.C., mother of a nine-year-old boy with Asperger's also felt, the first time her son's preschool suggested that something was wrong, that the real problem was the out-of-whack expectations being placed upon him. "His first day of school was 9/11. He fell down and cut his chin beforehand and needed stitches. School didn't take. After one morning the teacher called, concerned about him. 'Something's not right,' she said. 'He's frustrated, banging his head on the ground.' He had started to talk the way autistic children do, repeating back what other people say, reversing pronouns, repeating lines from movies and TV. The school sat me down and said he has sensory integration dysfunction. I felt the school was attempting to pathologize young behavior that was a little different."

Often, it took some kind of extreme shock to the system—behavior so bizarre that it couldn't be explained away by circumstances—to make a parent see that problems that had been present for years really had to be addressed. Sometimes, there was an incident that just pushed a parent over the edge, something that screamed at them, *Something has to be done.*

There were stories like this:

> *"When my daughter was about ten, one day, I served dinner on these little plates we had. She had been really hungry before dinner and I served the dinner and she said, 'You know, I'm really not hungry anymore.' Then it sort of struck me that she wouldn't eat off these plates.*
>
> *"I said, 'I will give you five dollars if you eat off that plate.' I said, 'I'll give you twenty dollars.' I said, 'I'll go to the bank and withdraw one hundred dollars if you'll eat off that plate,' and she burst into tears. She just couldn't eat off the plate. She couldn't touch the kitchen counter. She was pulling her eyebrows out."*

And like this:

> *"Something was different about my son from about two or three on. He just had so much separation anxiety. He'd go crazy if I left the room. He never matured out of it. I could never go to school for a field trip or with cupcakes because when I'd leave he'd cry for hours.*
>
> *"Then I had an epiphany one morning. We were getting ready for school. I couldn't find his usual shoes. So I took another pair. He became hysterical. I thought he was being difficult. I said, 'Honey, these shoes are perfectly good.' I said, 'Why does everything have to be so difficult with you?'*
>
> *"He said, 'Mommy, you don't understand. If I don't wear the other shoes, you're going to die today.'"*

For the Los Angeles mother, the tipping point was when her son's teacher took her aside one day and said, "Your child cannot focus." "She brought him over and sat him down and showed him his work and said, 'Can you finish anything in class and focus on anything?' He put his head down and said, 'No.' It was really painful for me to see him say, 'No, I can't.' That's when I said maybe I need to be a bit more flexible."

The parents I spoke with who ultimately decided to take their children in for treatment weren't looking at "normal" behavior—temper tantrums, less-than-optimal grades. "It's not 'normal boy' behavior for a five-year-old to frequently lash out at his parents in reaction to their constant criticism of his inability, or, in their view, his unwillingness, to conform to a reasonable level of domestic compliance," the parent of a boy with ADHD wrote in, angered by reader responses to my 2007 *New York Times* column "Ritalin Wars." "It's not 'normal boy' behavior to be smart yet unable to read for more than a few minutes when you're in second grade, and to be cruelly teased by your classmates, and chided by your teacher, for it. It's not 'normal boy' behavior to verbally whack your fifth-grade teacher who's riding you too hard for things you just can't control."

They weren't fiddling with the rough edges of growth or trying to get their kids to outperform their neighbors.

On the contrary: "My kids' issues have allowed me in part to just say no to competitive parenting," the Washington, D.C., mother of a severely depressed boy and a girl who struggles with anxiety, depression, and anorexia nervosa told me. "I can't compete in that mothering parade and my kids can't compete there. It's just got to go on without us."

These parents were trying to keep their kids at home. And in school.

"My child cannot get through a day," the mother of an adopted child with a prior history of abuse and neglect wrote in to the *Times*.

> *"Before medication she had crying jags that went on for as long as twelve or fourteen hours, during which she would sometimes go into a*

dissociative state. Risperdal has given her a life. . . . Strattera [a non-stimulant ADHD medication] controls her impulsivity (no, she cannot do that herself) and allows her to be in a classroom with normal children. The meds do NOT make her an easy child to deal with. They make her function and nothing more.

"Do people really think that I made these choices lightly? I went to many different doctors and fought the medications for a year. We tried changes in diet. I am well aware of the known and unknown consequences of the meds. But what else can I do? She is in therapy (frequently) but therapy only goes so far with a young child with low intelligence. Her parents and sibs all go to therapy to learn how to deal with her. Basically, we're doing all we can. In the good old days, before meds, she would have to have been institutionalized. With the meds, she will be a productive member of society."

In some cases, these parents were trying to keep their kids alive. This, at least, was the case of the D.C. mother I mentioned who commented on the competitive "mothering parade." Her daughter, an eleventh-grader at the time that we spoke, had been sensitive and irritable since birth. In fifth and sixth grade she'd been bullied badly in school and had developed Crohn's disease, a chronic, often extremely painful, inflammatory bowel disease. She also started having panic attacks and severe separation anxiety. The problems grew much worse when she began high school. She became anorexic.

"Freshman year, her panic and anxiety came back," her mother recalled. "I've struggled with depression, [my son] has had bouts of depression. I've never seen anything like this. We spent five months terrified that we'd turn around and she'd have done something to herself. She became incapacitated with anxiety, depression, and poor body image.

"We tried a variety of SSRIs and she had horrible reactions. She was jittery, jumpy. She fell into rubbing herself until her skin was raw. She'd

> *sit at the dining table crying for hours on end, blood coming through her socks. I understand why people in previous centuries believed in posession.*
>
> *"She really fell apart last year during spring break. She would have been hospitalized but she had such severe separation anxiety; she would sleep on top of me, wrap her hands in my shirt and walk around the house with me. The medical team decided against it. She didn't make it back to school for the rest of the year. We came close to losing her."*

"Now," she said, "she's on a terrible cocktail of Risperdal and antianxiety medications." Her daughter's not out of the woods, by a long shot. But she's able to leave the house every day to attend school.

The long march toward treatment often followed endless repetitions of teacher meetings and doctor appointments, testing, retesting, diagnosis and rediagnosis, false leads, bad advice, and, very often, useless half-measures, all of which left parents feeling powerless and afraid, and left children, sometimes, going years before receiving "help" that really did help.

Very often—though not always, and not exclusively—it was medication that helped. Yet the medications weren't a panacea. Often enough, they didn't work. Or they had terrible side effects: Stimulants brought on violent mood swings and atypical antipsychotics caused dangerous weight gains. "A granola bar would break and he would shriek and cry as the meds would wear off," the Los Angeles mother, who ultimately agreed, on and off, to put her son on medication, said. "At two months on Strattera, he was on an emotional roller coaster again, to the point that if he got upset he would bang his head against the wall."

Whenever they could, the parents tried to stop medication. In general, they let years go by before they were willing to even start medication. They tried everything else first: psychotherapy, vision therapy, auditory retraining, sensory integration therapy, biofeedback, energy work, acupuncture, nutritional counseling, friendship skills groups, martial arts training, magnetic pillows, yoga, vitamins, wheat-free diets, herbs. They called their lives, their parenting, themselves, deeply into question. When they could afford to, they cut back on work. They focused in more intently on their children. They made helping their children get better the central obsession of their lives.

Giving in to using medication very often felt like a mark of personal failure.

"We always think that we're going to be the couple that's different because, over the years, my husband has more often been the stay-at-home parent, the hands-on parent," a professor in southern Virginia told me. Even though she and her husband both had a history of depression—in the husband's case, it was chronic, and required sustained antidepressant use—they both believed that, by breaking the parenting mold, by doing everything right, setting up an optimally connected and nurturing home, they could inoculate their daughter against similar problems.

But then, when their daughter was in middle school, came a rude awakening. Their daughter became depressed. In high school, she suddenly started worrying about locking the doors. "In the summer of 2005, when she was fifteen," her mother said, "she was very nervous about noises in the house and made a particular effort to see that the doors were locked and the shades were down every night. This continued into the fall.

> *"It was starting to be a problem because it was taking an hour to lock three doors every night. We were starting to have words about it: 'You don't have to do that.' 'Yes I do.' She was loosening the locks—she was tugging on them so much. It was a ritualistic thing; there was a chanting thing. She was saying things to the doors as she locked them and checked them.*
>
> *"It was really unnerving. She's bright; she's funny; she's just a terrific kid and it looked just crazy. She was aware of that. We talked*

> *about it. I suggested going back to the therapist she'd seen before [for her depression].*
>
> *"She broke down, saying, 'I don't want to go see someone who says I have OCD because they'll make me stop what I'm doing, and I can't stop what I'm doing because I have to keep us safe."*

The girl did eventually start therapy, and was in addition treated with an SSRI antidepressant. Medication brought an "almost immediate improvement" to her symptoms, the mom said. But the parents didn't feel much better.

"My husband has over the years said, 'I feel like a chemistry experiment,'" the mom told me. "It's one thing to be one yourself, but another to make your child one. We felt like we'd failed. We felt somehow like we screwed up and that's why this was happening."

Giving a child psychotropic medication goes deeply against the grain for most parents. Medication is a mark of a lack of control, a definitive sign that a parent can't, through unconditional love or goodwill or connection or attachment or structure, create a perfect universe that will prevent his or her child's illness or disorder.

"We live the kind of life that most lay people believe would 'cure' ADD," a mother wrote to the *Times*.

> *"We're highly educated parents who manage to raise our children with only a few hours of high quality outside help each week. We live in a small town with nearly unlimited opportunities for unstructured outside play. Our children eat balanced, organic meals and are limited to three hours or less of extracurricular classes each week. We don't allow television during the week and severely limit it on the weekends. Every elementary teacher assigned to our children has had at least fifteen years of experience and possesses a specialized graduate degree. Despite a life full of the 'right' things, our son still can't function at school without Strattera."*

When medication proves itself able to do oceans more than you can do, it hurts. It gives a cold finality to the fact—so easy to avoid, to obfuscate, to rationalize away—that a child has serious problems.

"At core it's this: I have a flawed kid and I don't want a flawed kid," a North Carolina mother told me.

These are all terribly painful things to admit. Most parents do all they can to avoid admitting them—at least at first. This, I think, in part explains why so many dads stonewall when they're first confronted with the idea that there could be something wrong with their kids. The pain of the suggestion—with the sense of failure it brings—leads to a kind of shutting down.

"The OCD was much harder on him," the southern Virginia mom told me of her husband. "He could not stand to see her acting—as he said—'crazy.'"

It also may explain why parents very often don't give their kids their prescribed medications, or express their ambivalence toward medication by undermedicating, or discontinuing medications their children have been prescribed, even when they work. Stimulant medication has been shown to be effective in reducing the symptoms of ADHD 70 to 80 percent of the time. Yet studies of parents of children with ADHD have shown that about one-third of parents refuse to treat their children with stimulant medication when they're advised to by a physician. Up to 75 percent of parents, even after they've filled a prescription for medication for their child, don't give it as prescribed. Indeed, research shows, the fear of being prescribed medication keeps many parents—African-American parents in particular—from seeking help for their children in the first place.

Out of distrust of doctors, out of fear of medication, out of a desire to control a child's problems with good intentions and more-than-perfect parenting, some parents end up witnessing, and tolerating, a pretty extreme degree of distress.

One story that a reader told on *The New York Times* website has always, painfully, illustrated this for me. She was the mother of a ten-year-old girl who'd been formally diagnosed with ADHD at age seven, and she wrote in to the *Times* after I published my "Second Thoughts" column, saying that she could "relate" to the stories I'd told of children who cried through homework, self-destructively played the role of the "weird kid" at school to preempt other kids' rejection of them, and expressed their despair by threatening suicide. "In our case, our daughter sobbed for weeks and begged us to run over her with our car, it was horrible," she wrote. "Now we monitor her carefully to try to stop any downward spiral before it gets too far along. We work with a therapist for the anxiety and other ADD issues."

Her daughter was a "borderline enough case" that a psychiatrist had said the parents could go either way on medication. The dad was dead-set against drugs. But the mother, each and every day, wondered.

> *"On one hand academically, she is fine because her grades are fine, straight As. But that is because she spends so much time on homework, at least twice as long as the other kids (due to slow processing speed and distractibility), and has to bring home work from school that she has not finished (too distracted in school), plus work on weekends. She does it—but there are lots of too-late nights, and the whole scene is very draining for all of us. . . . If she doesn't get the grades that match her intelligence, she is devastated. . . .*
>
> *"She is in pain, I know it. We try to give her as much support as we possibly can. . . .*
>
> *"My daughter is a beautiful, brilliant girl. I so hope we are doing right by her."*

Another mother, in New Hampshire, described to me how, living in the woods, off the grid, with only organic food to eat and no TV, she had tried to create the healthiest possible home for her children. She'd worked as few hours as possible, homeschooled them, and tried to be "the perfect mother: someone who never lost her temper and was always available, able to not only listen but to understand," she said.

Yet, despite all that, her daughter developed black rages at age fourteen. She had violent outbursts and mood swings so dramatic that when her mood went down "the whole house would feel filled with her unhappiness," the mother told me. She said her daughter started to remind her of two of her own sisters: "We have a history of mental illness in my family," she said. But, no matter how bad things got, she still did not take her daughter for help. "I was feeling like I should be able to handle this and there was some shame that I couldn't," she said.

Ultimately, the girl moved away, choosing to finish high school while living with an aunt in Tucson, Arizona. She eventually found a therapist, was diagnosed with depression, and after some unsuccessful rounds with antidepressants ended up in a psych ward, where, at age nineteen, she was diagnosed as bipolar and put on effective medication.

"There's so much self-blame for me," her mother says now. "I did my best. I don't think any of us do everything right."

Who can blame the parents who let their children suffer undiagnosed and untreated? Who can imagine how hard it is to make the decision to seek mental health services for a kid at a time when everyone and everything is warning you about rampant overdiagnosis and the perfidy of medication?

The idea that, through sheer force of will, you can control your child's every experience, create a perfect environment, and guarantee him or her the right kind of life, is the core belief of the parenting culture that reigns in our time. It is one of the great points of uniqueness of parents of children with mental health issues that they are forced—long before others—to learn the fallacy of that dogma.

"I was on the playground once when my son had not yet been diagnosed but was just in speech therapy," a Washington, D.C., mother with a seven-year-old boy who has Asperger's (and, uncharacteristically for Asperger's, had a speech delay) told me. "I saw these other parents pushing their children on the swings and having their very little girl recite the alphabet. And I realized that they think, *They did this*. Parents of normal children have this conceit that if your child has one of these labels, you screwed up and you're just looking for an excuse. A lot of random stuff happens and people don't realize it. You invest so much in your children and you sacrifice so much and you have to acknowledge that you don't have control."

I believe that the combination of avoidance and a desire for control explains in part, why, in the face of unanimous disagreement from mainstream scientists, parents cling to debunked ideas about the causes of mental disorders—that excess sugar causes ADHD, for example, or that vaccines cause autism. You can eliminate sugar; you can, however foolishly, refuse to vaccinate your child. These factors also, I think, explain why, in an age where mental health professionals themselves no longer blame parents, mothers and fathers continue to beat themselves up for their children's mental disorders. If you're guilty, after all, you can try to set things right—you have some modicum of power and control.

Lisa Carver, the mother of a schizophrenic boy who sometimes receives "messages" from caterpillars that cry out to him to save them, addresses this issue head-on in her essay, "My Other Half," in the 2007 anthology *The Elephant in the Playroom*. "If his behavior were your fault," she writes, "then you could work to change it."

Misguided guilt—plus the belief that there *must* be a fixable cause for a child's symptoms—I now believe causes the kinds of "crazy"-seeming parental behaviors I once saw, without comprehension, around me in Washington, D.C., and that inspired the first (mis)conception of this book. I saw, without seeing, parents whose very young children were starting to show signs of disorders like Asperger's, ADHD, and learning disabilities. They ran from therapy to therapy, tried diet after diet, radiated an extreme form of the control-freakishness so rampant in our world because, I now understand, they wanted mastery, to help, to *do something.*

The "quest for a cause," Boston-area pediatricians Perri Klass and Eileen Costello write in *Quirky Kids: Understanding and Helping Your Child Who Doesn't Fit In,* can for many parents easily become "a mission, even an obsession." When it leads to unproven remedies like chelation—a chemical treatment some parents try in an attempt to "cure" their children's autism by removing heavy metals from their bodies—it can be downright dangerous.

At some point, a number of the parents I spoke with came to feel that their own issues were getting in the way of helping their children. Some ultimately learned that, in order to get their children's problems under control, they actually had to relinquish control, or give up on the forms of control they'd been trying to use before. This, at least, was the conclusion reached by a woman in rural Maryland whose family life had been taken over by her son's extreme impulsivity and restlessness before he was treated for ADHD.

"He was always breaking things and throwing things. He was in constant motion. He had no concept of consequences—they meant nothing to him. I can't tell you how many times he ran in front of cars. It got to where we didn't go to friends' houses," she recalled of the early years of her now nineteen-year-old son's life.

> *"I just couldn't relax. I couldn't take him to stores because he'd run away. We had a number of babysitters—he'd lock them out of the house, chase them with knives, bite or kick them. Normally, you can sit*

down with a kid and explain things. With him you couldn't; he'd be off running.

"I was yelling at him all the time. I yelled and I screamed. I did that because I didn't want to hit him. In school, in baseball or football, the kids were picking on him to see his reaction. He was always in trouble, always getting sent to the principal's office. . . .

"My husband and I tried desperately then not to put him on medication. We tried the Feingold diet—no artificial colors, flavors, preservatives. We read every book. Every time we heard of a natural remedy, we tried it. I didn't want to pop a pill in his mouth; I don't like to take pills. I wanted to try everything humanly possible before medication.

"One day my husband said something that got to me: 'He needs it for him, not for you.'"

The Los Angeles mom put off giving her son medication just as long as she could. She pushed for school accommodations, and met with her son's teacher weekly. She hired an educational therapist. She tried homeopathy, martial arts, brain-training software, biofeedback—anything she could.

But after the confrontation with her son's fourth-grade teacher, she cracked. "We tried a low dose of Ritalin—just the word sounds so evil," she told me.

"My son said, 'My brain is like a chameleon. You know, chameleons have eyes that don't look straight ahead—that's how my brain is. But when I take the vitamins'—that's what we called the Ritalin—'my eyes look straight ahead.' The chameleon image—it's hard to refute that. If your kid has chameleon eyes, it's really hard to tell him to make them go straight ahead."

She reacted to Ritalin's effectiveness with something less than jubilation.

"I decided not to say anything to the teacher," she said. "The first day I gave him Ritalin, I bumped into her. She said, 'You know what, it's amazing. We had a fabulous day.' I wanted to burst out crying. You want this thing not to work."

I heard this repeatedly from parents of children for whom medication actually worked: sadness, regret, a ruefulness bordering almost on resentment.

"One little pill, and he's a different kid," a New York mother said to me mournfully, after ADHD medication changed her sixth-grader's homework time from a four-hour screamfest to a peaceful and productive hour and a half.

It was as though, if the meds worked, then there really was something wrong. A child's issue wasn't just a passing problem. The parents were in it for the long haul. If not for life.

· 5 ·

Who, Exactly, Is Having Issues?

"People are so stressed out, and it's so much easier to say, 'Here, take this pill and go to your room; leave me alone.'"

LISA POPCZYNSKI, WHO CHOSE BEHAVIORAL THERAPY OVER MEDICATION FOR HER TEN-YEAR-OLD SON WITH ADHD, TO *THE NEW YORK TIMES*, DECEMBER 22, 2006

"I suffered from ADHD that was not diagnosed until my son began exhibiting the same symptoms," a woman named Sue wrote to *The New York Times* as part of the heady reader response that followed the publication of my "Second Thoughts" change-of-heart column.

"'Suffered' is an accurate term," she continued. "I was ridiculed by peers, teachers, and even family members for my lack of organizational skills, verbal impulsivity, and difficulty concentrating. These were all interpreted as laziness and passive-aggressive behavior."

She learned to live with the criticism. She learned to work around her difficulties. She succeeded in becoming a clinical psychologist. "But," she wrote, "the social and emotional costs were immeasurable."

When her son started to have similar difficulties in school, Sue opposed putting him on medication. She believed in the power of psychotherapy, she wrote. "I was convinced that the pressures of modern urban life, the paucity of outlets for excess physical energy, and the chemicals in fast food were major contributors to so many kids' symptoms."

In the end, however, the strength of her beliefs and the efforts she made to build an ideal world for her son weren't sufficient to save him from the pain she herself had known as a girl and young woman. She had, she decided, to give medication a go.

"I would love for all of us to live in an ideal village, with plenty of emotional and material support for every family; a twenty-hour work week; fresh, organic food that is easily available and affordable . . . and [where] spontaneous creative thinking and behavior was rewarded and not ridiculed and repressed," she wrote.

> *"We don't live there, though. Our family, like most, struggles to pay the bills and accomplish everything we need to do to get through to tomorrow. . . . My son has professional ambitions that he is capable of fulfilling, but not if he flunks his classes because he chronically forgets and loses assignments. Would I love to send him to a nurturing private school where he might be able to accomplish these things unmedicated? Sure. In fact, we did go the private route for a while, living in cramped, substandard housing, working overtime, and forgoing vacations and restaurant meals to pay tuition (and were criticized then for not spending enough time supervising his homework or planning recreational activities), but he suffered there as well.*
>
> *"He, and I, are doing much better on a low dose of stimulant medication. It's not ideal, and we don't take the possible side effects lightly. But my sensitive, loving, 'intellectually superior' kid is now managing to pass his courses and get through most days without being ridiculed and bullied for his 'weirdness.' It's better than what I had, though I wish I could do better for him."*

I don't know why it is that parents like this—with their complicated, ambiguous stories, their ambivalence, their guilt and pain—haven't dominated, or even made a dent in, the coverage of the issue of children and meds. Instead, the grasping, grade-mongering, irresponsible, selfish, pushy parent is the archetype that dominates the public imagination, inspiring headlines like "Parents Push the New Abnormal," and giving people the sense that parents are "drugging" their kids for their own ease and convenience, and as an antidote to their own incompetence.

I never once, in the course of the five years I spent researching and writing this book, met a pushy parent who blithely medicated his or her kid, piling on more and more drugs to better control bad or suboptimal behavior. As I indicated in the last chapter, these parents don't appear, statistically, really to exist in any significant numbers. What research there is shows that parents don't like psychiatric drugs, don't want to use them, and frequently undermedicate their kids, even when they've ostensibly accepted the idea of drug treatment. In fact, most parents don't get their kids with issues any mental health care at all.

In the course of my research, I met only one parent who said she'd been eager (or, in retrospect, thought of herself as having been eager) to put her child on medication. She was the mother of a boy who in preschool had always been in trouble. He was disruptive, hyperemotional, aggressive to other kids. The boy's pediatrician, without any formal evaluation, suggested a trial of ADHD meds. The medication made the boy all but psychotic. At age five, he was talking about suicide.

The mother stopped the drugs and took the boy to see a child psychiatrist. The psychiatrist diagnosed him as bipolar on the spot—based on his reaction to the ADHD meds. (Many children end up being diagnosed as bipolar—and end up on bipolar meds—after becoming manic or violent or psychotic or otherwise out of control on stimulant medication or SSRI antidepressants.)

The mom went home and read up on the side effects and dangers of the bipolar meds. And she threw her prescription away. She reduced her working hours. She got her son some intensive therapy. She put him in an all boys' school where there was plenty of time in the day for running around, playing sports, and otherwise blowing off steam. His school behavior improved greatly.

"He's not out of the woods," she told me years later. "He's still got some issues." She talked about his anxiety and hypersensitivity. It was, she said, his genetic inheritance; his dad had these issues, too.

Looking ahead, she anticipated that the family was still in for some serious challenges. Looking back to her son's preschool days, she judged herself sharply. "Believe me, if there was a pill that would have taken all that trouble away, I would have jumped at it," she said.

Except that, when push came to shove, she really hadn't.

Some doctors have played a big role in making the lazy-irresponsible-pill-pushing-parent stereotype seem real. Northern California child psychiatrist Elizabeth J. Roberts, for one, painted a damning portrait of such parents in a 2006 op-ed for *The Washington Post*. "These days parents cruise the Internet, take self-administered surveys, diagnose their children and choose a medication before they ever set foot in the psychiatrist's office," she wrote. "If the first doctor doesn't prescribe what you want, the next one will."

The National Institute of Mental Health's Daniel Pine did parents no favor either when he spelled out a very real-sounding "hypothetical example" of performance-mad parenting for George Washington University anthropologist Roy Richard Grinker.

"A mother and a father bring their twelve-year-old son to you because, as they report it, 'he is doing poorly' at an exclusive private school with a demanding curriculum. When you look at the boy's transcript you notice that the boy received mostly grades of B. Teachers report that he is somewhat fidgety, doesn't pay attention quite as often as other kids, and sometimes seems irritable, but they don't say he's disruptive, outside the norm, or in need of any kind of educational or cognitive assessment. He just isn't an A student," he mused, for Grinker's 2007 book, *Unstrange Minds:*

> *"And the parents are pushing you to do something, and they even bring up the subject of medication by themselves, and they know all the criteria for ADHD, and they've read books and have been all over the Internet on this thing. They've read some new article you haven't even seen. And so maybe you medicate him, and to medicate him and have insurance reimburse for it, you give a diagnosis of ADHD, and suddenly you've got a kid with this label. See how easy it can happen?"*

It is easy, I guess, hypothetically. And yet, when I interviewed doctors—including Pine—to see how frequently this sort of thing really happened to them, they were hard-pressed to come up with much by way of real experience.

There are *some* parents, I was told, who truly are too eager to try medication, in part to avoid looking at problems in their own lives. "There are parents who really do look to pin all the problems on something that's wrong with the child, because it's easier for them, it takes less time, they're self-involved, selfish, caught up in work, not willing to put in the time to look at what's going on in the family. Usually in those cases there are family issues and there are conduct issues," a psychologist in Virginia who specializes in attention and anxiety disorders told me. But, he said, those parents were, in his experience, "very rare."

"I don't know who these parents are, these lazy, neglectful parents," ADHD specialist and *Driven to Distraction* coauthor Edward M. Hallowell put it to me more bluntly. "I've not met them. I think they're a fiction. I see parents who are working full-time and also trying to do their best for their children."

When I went back to a couple of the doctors who'd been very vocal, in print, about making it sound like every free-spirited Tom Sawyer and Pippi Longstocking (to paraphrase Northern California behavioral pediatrician Larry Diller) was being pumped full of drugs, their views of parents were a lot more nuanced than their sound bites let on. Diller himself, for example, who had infamously written, "I, in my role as specialist, do this all the time—medicate children with drugs like Ritalin, Adderall, and Prozac, much more frequently than I care to—even when I feel they have *nothing seriously wrong with them*," in his 2006 book, *The Last Normal Child*, expressed sympathy for parents.

"I don't know any parent who jumps at the idea of medicating their kid," he told me.

Daniel Pine, when I looked him up to find out whether his "hypothetical" was based on truth, responded to my question much like the parents I challenged when they told me "all" the kids they knew were on meds.

He shut me down.

"You're quoting me out of context," he said.

I read the passage in Grinker's book back to him in its entirety.

"The context is the pressure people feel to make the diagnosis," he said. "There's a lot of pressure on the practitioner to not get caught up in the pressure to do something and fix something," he said.

"Does this ever happen to you?" I asked.

"Personally, I would not prescribe a treatment for a child with any psychiatric disorder unless I thought that was what was going on," he answered.

Had this happened to *anyone* Pine knew firsthand?

"I've never heard of anything like that on the one hand," he said. He then added, "On the other hand, it's very common to talk to physicians who struggle with what to do. All the clinicians I know would say they do the best they can to form a diagnosis first and then prescribe a treatment."

So—"all" kids are on meds—except they're not.

"Parents" are shoving pills down their children's throats for their own ease and convenience—except they're not.

"Doctors" are complicit in this—except they're not.

Why is it so hard to find real people who fit these stereotypes? And more curious still, why do the stereotypes—these "hypothetical people"—seem so real?

After puzzling over these questions for some time, it dawned on me, late in writing this book, that there might be a rather simple explanation for at least part of the mystery. All the doctors whom I'd seen quoted, or had interviewed, about pushy parents overdrugging their kids practiced in wealthy areas. And while these doctors might not literally have been seeing parents coming in begging for meds, they were routinely seeing mothers and fathers who were obsessed with their children's status and performance, as parents in upper-middle-class communities across the country often tend to be.

These parents are not necessarily the most endearing people. Their expectations can be grandiose; their sense of entitlement can be grating; their ability to purchase the best of everything for their kids can be poisonously envy-inspiring.

I could imagine how easy it would be for doctors in well-off communities to come to think the very worst of the parents whom they saw day after day. I could also see how easy it would be for them to believe that their observations and experiences were similar to those of all parents, and doctors, in our competitive, high-pressure era. ("Virtually all parents seem to feel that their child has an inner A-student waiting to be revealed, if only he could sit down and do his homework," a pediatrician in an "affluent suburb," glibly generalized to the *Times,* explaining online that he "almost daily" saw parents asking if their child's "academic mediocrity" could be attributed to ADHD.)

That sort of conflation, that kind of generalization, is what the news media has done all the time in recent years, while covering the story of pushy parents pathologizing their kids. So much so that, in the public mind, the story of wealthy parents misusing children's mental health services and of other parents trying to simply procure mental health services have become inextricably intertwined.

Think of all the stories of high school parents pressuring neuropsychologists to test and label their kids as "learning disabled" in order to earn extra time on the SAT. (One Bay Area educational psychologist told the *San Francisco Chronicle* back in 2003 that she'd started demanding payment up front for her services, because some parents, if test results *didn't* show an accommodation-enabling learning disability, were refusing to pay.) Remember the "anxiety industry" of preschooler test prep for private kindergartens in New York City. The parents in wealthy Westport, Connecticut, suing their school district to get reimbursement for "special-education" services like horseback riding and personal trainers.

All of these stories have led to a perception that a lot of the treatments and services related to children's mental health—whether meds, therapy, special education, or school accommodations—are basically a sham, a way for some parents to help their kids get a leg up on everyone else. "At elite high schools and colleges around the country," conservative commentator Mary Eberstadt claimed in her 2004 book, *Home-Alone America*, "'learning disabled' is broadly understood to be synonymous with 'educational scam.'"

The pervasiveness of this view hasn't made things particularly pleasant for parents of kids with learning disabilities or other special mental health needs.

"There are people who see us as an abuse of the system," a mother in Fairfax, Virginia, whose ten-year-old son had been receiving free care from the state since he was diagnosed with Asperger's syndrome at age two and a half, told me.

Her son, she said, had made great strides, thanks to those early intervention services. Such great strides that it isn't always obvious to outsiders that he's still on the autistic spectrum or needs special services, particularly since he gets perfect scores on standardized tests. His brother has ADHD, takes medication, and is able to hold his own in his school's gifted and talented program.

This hasn't, the mom explained, made the family very popular with the neighbors.

"One kid in G&T, ostensibly getting a better education, and the other getting support. . . . People look at that like, *You really know how to work the system*," she said bitterly. "There's a lot of *unrest*, let's say."

The unrest is understandable. Times being so tough for so many, there's really no underestimating the amount of envy and resentment that circulates today among parents. It's very easy to see one child's gain as another child's loss, particularly since parents really are competing for resources in our public school systems.

Special ed, after all, is mandated by a federal law, the Individuals with Disabilities Education Act, which guarantees all children, regardless of disability, the right to a "free, appropriate" education. It is paid for locally, however, and has never been properly funded. In recent decades, as the number of students receiving services has gone up and up (along with more and better diagnosis), school-system budgets have not kept pace, and as money has continually been diverted toward special-ed students, it has been drained away from all the rest.

It can cost up to $150,000 a year to educate a child with extreme special needs. If parents can prove that their district's public schools can't provide appropriate services for their child, then local taxpayer funds may be used to pay for private school. This fact can be particularly enraging for parents who can't afford private school for their own kids and are less than thrilled with their public options. Like Washington,

D.C., parents who in 2006 learned that slightly over 2,000 special-ed students—4 percent of the beleaguered system's enrollment—were attending private schools at public expense, and were consuming 15 percent of the city's education budget. Or New York City parents who in 2007 learned that former Viacom chief executive Tom Freston—who'd left his company with a golden parachute worth $85 million—was asking the New York City public school system to reimburse his son's $37,900-a-year tuition at a private school for children with learning disabilities.

Freston's story got great play. However outrageous—and unusual—his own situation, it was easy to portray it as just the tip of an iceberg of parental scheming and corruption. (New York City education officials did this eagerly, as they refused Freston's demand, and the case made its way through the courts.) For the idea that a small, rich minority of people is reaping unfair advantages for themselves and their children is one of the overarching fears—and truths—of our time.

And the perception that it's the kids from the wealthiest homes who get the most diagnoses and the most, and best, services, isn't false.

The most competitive schools often show disproportionate numbers of students with learning disabilities.The most affluent school districts across the country do register the greatest numbers of children getting special accommodations in school and extra time on the SATs.

All these facts lend themselves easily to the accusation that wealthy parents are gaming the system to get even greater advantages for their kids. Some, as the *San Francisco Chronicle*'s educational psychologist made clear, surely are. But for the most part, this odd situation reflects a much larger and darker reality: Only parents with considerable means (and the time and the savvy that usually accompany such means) are able to work our school systems to get the services and accommodations to which kids with issues are entitled.

It's very hard, if you don't have copious amounts of time and money, to sue a school system to get private education reimbursed for a special-needs child. As Daniel Golden wrote in *The Wall Street Journal* in July

2007, lawyers are expensive and the legal hurdles are considerable. Before bringing a suit, parents have to pass through administrative review hearings, presided over by hearing officers who are typically trained or hired by state education departments and generally rule for the school districts. In recent years, in an effort to control costs, courts have tended to side even more often with school districts, and Congress has amended the disabilities law to greatly increase the legal and financial burden on parents. As a result, the number of hearings in recent years has begun to drop, as are taxpayer-funded placements in private schools.

Even the basic special-education services that public school districts are legally required to provide for children with learning or other issues are very difficult to access for parents without time and considerable energy and resources. The Individuals with Disabilities Education Act, or IDEA, created a process whereby children with special needs were entitled to have an "individual education plan" created for them, which was intended to provide them with the best possible education in the "least restrictive environment." The IEP was to be created by a team of teachers, administrators, social workers, and psychologists, and agreed to by parents. If the participants in the IEP process didn't agree, either side had the right to demand a formal hearing. If that didn't resolve the dispute, either side could bring suit in federal court.

The process is complicated and confusing—and expensive, if it goes to court—and scares off many poor and working-class parents. Not surprisingly, the parents most likely to get good IEPs for their children are the wealthiest and most sophisticated. Having a nonworking spouse in the family—a person who can make pursuing a child's educational rights a full-time occupation—also tends to be a necessary precondition of getting the system to work.

The experiences of the parents I interviewed illustrated this sorry situation perfectly.

One mother, an affluent former lawyer in Texas, who has a background in special education and neuroscience and now stays home full-time with her kids, fought tooth and nail against her Dallas school district when she began to see signs that her young son had some kind of learning disability.

He had been tested and scored high in intelligence. Yet he was struggling to learn to read and "hated sitting down to write."

Because he was managing to work at grade level, he was denied the right to be tested by the school and to receive special-education services. "A teacher would look at him and say, 'He's lazy,'" she told me.

The mom knew dyslexia when she saw it. She also knew, from her special-ed work, that Texas had passed a law in 1985 requiring its school districts to proactively identify and tutor children with dyslexia. She knew—unlike most parents in the state—that to get help she had to request a special-ed evaluation; it wouldn't be forthcoming from the school. She had no trouble demanding it. And she had the time, and the training, to persevere. She got the evaluation, which showed her son was dyslexic. She proved to school officials that they were misinterpreting state law by denying him services just because he wasn't failing. "I had to be the expert. I read them the law," she told me. "They were just perceiving me as nuts."

And, in the end, she got her son the specialized tutoring he needed.

Most parents don't have that kind of time and expertise. A full-time working mother in Maryland with a high school–level education also suspected that her son had learning issues and that his school wasn't doing enough to get him help. He was smart, he was motivated, but he had a terrible time learning to read.

"When he was little, I kept telling him someday he's going to invent something that will save people's lives, but he just had this reading problem," the mother told me. "When he was first tested, the people said we've never seen a kid like this; on the one hand, he's a genius, and on the other, he's the total opposite. They identified a memory problem they couldn't name."

The only accommodation the boy received from his school for the learning disability was extra time on tests. As time passed, his mother had to give up on her dream that, unlike her husband and herself, her son would attend college.

Now nineteen, he works two part-time jobs with no benefits. His parents have seen ads for jobs at the post office and encouraged him to consider them, but he won't apply: "It means taking a test," she said.

"We considered getting him private tutoring, but money was a factor," the mother remembered of her son's elementary school years. "Where we live there aren't that many people doing it. He's the fourth of four boys. . . ." Her voice trailed off. "It's probably not an excuse."

A Washington, D.C., mother who'd battled her neighborhood public school to get proper testing and accommodations for her son had a story that was fairly typical, too. Her son's kindergarten and first-grade years had been ones of constant struggle, discipline issues, miscommunication, and frustration.

"He didn't sit still. His performance in class was not what standardized tests indicated it ought to be and not what it was if he was alone. Handwriting was very difficult for him. He was breaking pencils all the time but was a different kid if he was writing on computers," his mom recalled. "We initiated the process to have him tested by [the D.C. public schools]," she said. "We couldn't afford private testing. It took a whole year of arguing, and we got nothing."

In third grade, the school finally tested him. The testing showed his IQ to be in the 120s, which is considered to be superior to very superior. School officials suggested then that he be labeled emotionally disturbed. She protested this—she didn't believe it was true and didn't want him shipped off to a school for emotionally disturbed kids. "Then," she said, "they tried to say he was retarded."

This mother had been forced to leave her job at a government agency after a car accident had left her in chronic pain. When, after a long wait, her workers' compensation payments came through, she was finally able to pay for private testing and hired an educational consultant to help her and her husband negotiate with the D.C. public schools. Private testing produced a diagnosis of ADHD and sensory integration issues. The educational consultant helped the family find a place for the boy at a private school that specialized in children with learning issues. The parents successfully sued the city for tuition reimbursement. At the new school, the boy began to thrive.

"By the end of the year, we were talking about a regular school for him. He had new coping skills for sensory integration and was doing fantastically," his mom told me. "By the end of fourth grade, he was doing sixth- to eighth-grade level work and had a twelfth-grade vocabulary," she said. "How do parents who aren't educated and obnoxious get anything done for their kids?"

As with so much else in our country, when it comes to mental health care, the affluent have access to wonderful things, including specialized dyslexia tutoring that actually retrains the brain; cognitive behavioral therapy that also rewires the brain and can bring enormous benefits to kids with anxiety, obsessive-compulsive disorder, and depression; social skills training for ADHD; and intensive speech and behavioral therapies that can lead some mildly autistic children to "recover" so dramatically that they can appear indistinguishable from other kids.

Everyone else, most often, gets absolutely nothing.

Hundreds of thousands of kids in Texas don't get special-ed services, a 2007 survey found, because the state just isn't doing its job in reaching out to identify them. (And, the same survey illustrated, in Houston, 70 percent of the identified dyslexic students were concentrated in the more affluent areas.)

The 2006 *Washington Post* story that reported 2,283 (generally affluent) special-education students were using taxpayer funds to attend private school also found that 2,521 children in the city were backlogged, awaiting services that had been officially ordered for them but never materialized. Lower-income parents who couldn't afford lawyers just couldn't shake the system hard enough to get out of it what their kids needed. And D.C.'s school system itself, the *Post* revealed, was profoundly chaotic, full of unqualified personnel and children stuck for years without any hope of ever getting appropriate services.

I heard more of this anecdotally as well. "I got this testing report once from the D.C. public schools that said this one kid was deaf," the former admissions director of a private special-ed school in the District told me. "He was blind in one eye—from an eye infection because he was from a family that just didn't have any resources—but he wasn't deaf."

In Georgia, in 2007, 85 percent of the families who applied for tuition vouchers under a new scholarship program aimed at helping special-ed students find more and better school options were unable to use their vouchers either because they couldn't find a school to accept their child, couldn't afford the additional costs of private school, or didn't satisfy the program's complex eligibility criteria.

On Long Island, a 2008 survey by *Newsday* found, affluent districts were labeling five times as many of their students as autistic as were poorer areas. The reason: New York State's push to expand special-education help for autistic children had pretty much entirely passed by those disadvantaged communities. Poorer children who were not being taken for regular pediatrician visits were not getting diagnosed early. And poor and minority children with autism were still being classified as mentally retarded.

Now that more children are being diagnosed than ever before with learning disabilities and other mental health needs, many states can't keep up with the demand for services. Nowhere is the problem more acute than in the vastly growing and expensive demand for autism-related services. In Massachusetts, where the number of schoolchildren diagnosed with autism nearly doubled between 2002 and 2007, special schools for autistic children have had to close their doors to new students. In Colorado, children are weeded out through intelligence testing: if their IQ proves to be over 70—a cutoff that excludes many of those with Asperger's and high-functioning autism—they don't qualify for state services at all.

Many states now have long waiting lists for special services. But developmental disorders like autism can't wait. Excellent private services exist, particularly in large urban areas, but they're ruinously expensive. Many health insurance companies won't cover autism services, or, if they do, they pay for it at the lower reimbursement rate used for other mental health services. As a result, parents of autistic children nationwide are bankrupting themselves paying privately for early intervention programs, speech therapy, and O.T. Parents of children with learning disabilities are spending their every last cent on private tutoring. Or—when they feel they have no choice—simply watching their kids grow up without services.

And when it comes to other sorts of mental health services, the story is the same.

Although it's popularly believed—in some circles, at least—that "all" kids are now either on meds or in therapy (even infants, *The Wall Street Journal* reported in 2006, noting that "therapists are increasingly moving their treatments from the couch to the crib"), the fact is that only 5 to 7 percent of children ever see a mental health specialist. Approximately 70 percent of children and teens who need mental health treatment don't receive any services at all.

Despite reports of an epidemic-level mental meltdown among today's college students, fewer than 25 percent of college-age Americans with mental health problems get treatment. Only 5 percent of young Americans with substance-abuse disorders get help. Only 9 percent of college students even try to get counseling services on campus. Those who do try often face long waits to see overburdened counselors. For troubled students in the University of California system, the wait to see a counselor in recent years was three to six weeks.

This is the truth about children's mental health care in America: For most kids, it's nonexistent. "The number of children with untreated mental illnesses is as high now as it was twenty years ago," an exhaustive National Institute of Mental Health report declared early in this decade; it called the "deficiencies" in mental health services for children in our country simply "staggering." Things haven't gotten any better.

There are only about seven thousand child psychiatrists currently practicing in our country, overwhelmingly concentrated in the big cities. Many have long waiting lists. In some rural areas, there are no child psychiatrists—or even child psychologists—at all.

Most children receive what services they do from their pediatricians. But many pediatricians now are loath to treat kids with mental disorders, fearful of deadly side effects from medications they were not specifically trained to prescribe, and unable to provide the time for proper follow-up. And research has shown that pediatricians are often unable to recognize mental health issues and frequently fail to refer kids with mental health needs to specialists. In North Carolina, one survey showed that only 2 percent of the children with significant emotional and behavioral disorders in the state were being seen by mental health specialists. The best-informed, best-intentioned pediatrician, after all, can't do a full psychiatric evaluation—which can last hours—in a typical eight- to twelve-minute consultation.

The American Academy of Child and Adolescent Psychiatry is currently working with the American Academy of Pediatrics to try to formalize ways to collaborate on caring for children with mental health needs, but models for such joint care are scarce. Some insurance companies won't reimburse pediatricians for time they spend providing mental health services. None are reimbursed for time spent on the phone trying to find or consult with a child psychiatrist.

Even when they do get referrals from pediatricians, families often fail to follow up when mental health services are recommended. Most, as I said before, are reluctant to give their children medication, and as a result prefer not to see med-prescribing psychiatrists. Most tend to believe more strongly in the benefits of therapy. But therapy, very often, is impossibly expensive. Most private health plans reimburse mental health services at much lower rates—and with much greater restrictions—than they do other medical needs. And more than half of all outpatient specialty mental health services for children with private insurance are provided out of plan.

Parents' refusal, or reluctance, to get their kids mental health care isn't entirely a matter of economics, though.

Psychologists Madeline Levine and Suniya Luthar have found many affluent parents to be uniquely resistant to seeking mental health care for their kids, for reasons that have nothing to do with money. Rather, they have found, what motivates these parents is a desire to save face. Wealthy parents, Luthar has written, feel even more compelled than other parents to maintain a "veneer of well-being" about their families. In addition, school psychologists often hesitate to express their concerns to wealthy parents out of a fear of push back and even lawsuits. In the end, Levine concludes in *The Price of Privilege*, "the children of the most affluent families are often the *least* likely to be referred for therapy."

African-American children are also particularly unlikely to receive mental health services.They're less likely than whites to be diagnosed with mental health issues when they exhibit problem behaviors at school. And despite the widespread perception that black children are being singularly pathologized—and singled out for the almost punitive use of meds, the truth is that they're far less likely than white kids to take medication. (One 2003 study showed white kids diagnosed with ADHD to be *nine times* as likely to receive a prescription for stimulant meds than were minority children, even when researchers controlled for age, gender, length of visit, and type of insurance coverage.)

As a result, minority children suffer disproportionately from the burden of untreated mental illness. They get less treatment, poorer treatment, and more punishment. Black children in particular are more likely to be viewed as "bad"—rather than impaired—by schools, doctors, and even their parents, determined a team of researchers exploring black-white differences in attitudes toward ADHD.

Rather than receive treatment, black children with ADHD and other mental health issues are disproportionately subjected to school disciplinary actions like suspensions and expulsions. This may be part of the reason why, nationwide, black students are suspended and expelled from school at nearly three times the rate of white students.

A North Carolina mother I interviewed was intimately acquainted with what it meant to struggle daily against a system that viewed her mentally ill son as "bad." Her son had been diagnosed with ADHD when he was five ("he became a Ritalin baby, which I resisted with all my heart, mind, and soul," she said), and was later diagnosed with depression so severe that he had to be hospitalized twice in his first year of high school.

"He's an African-American male. I'm a single mom," she began.

> *"He has emotional problems, but many people don't differentiate: they say, 'You act like this because of the color of your skin.' They say, 'You're angry, you're threatening to me.' But he's responding with a tone of voice that indicates frustration, not anger. The school system was not equipped in terms of counselors, of not wanting to hear his history, not wanting to deal with a kid outside of certain parameters.*
>
> *"He was suspended from school a few times for perceived threats. Before one suspension, he and a white boy were talking in class and*

> *talking back to the teacher—an older white female teacher. The white boy was said to be 'disruptive.' My son was 'disrespectful and threatening.' He was suspended, the other boy was not."*

"Provider bias," a tendency among doctors and school psychologists to view African-American children more as victims, or vectors, of social pathology than of mental illness, is part of the story of why so many black children in need of help go undiagnosed and untreated. But to a large degree, undertreatment is also due to a profound distrust of psychologists, psychiatrists, and "helping professionals" generally on the part of black parents, for many of whom the idea of having a child singled out or labeled carries a potent sting of stigma and condemnation.

I heard this pain strongly in the voice of a mother in Dallas, who'd been profoundly hurt when a teacher had suggested that her daughter might have ADHD.

"Last year, I received a note from the kindergarten teacher saying she wanted to speak to me about my daughter," she told me. "The teacher said, 'She seems like she's in her own world. She has pretend friends. I really think you need to talk to her pediatrician about getting her on some kind of drug because she's not focused, is distracting the other kids.'"

"She separated my daughter from the other students," she continued, her voice cracking with emotion. "She put her desk next to hers. I felt, *What have I done?* The teacher was saying there is something mentally wrong with my daughter. I didn't want to go to the pediatrician," she continued.

> *"I'm African-American. There are certain things that some of us do not want to take on directly. Like going to a psychiatrist when there's a problem. We try instead to work it out on our own. It's just the stereotype that's placed on it—that you're crazy, not doing it right. The fear of being accused of something that's not true. The drugs out there for ADD—you hear stories of what they do to children. I'm a single mother*

and when you hear things like this, you panic. We say, 'No—we can handle it in our own way.'"

Today's biological psychiatry—with its emphasis on inherited disorders—can be inherently problematic for a group that has suffered, over the generations, from "expert" beliefs about their genetic inferiority. Psychology, too, is often perceived as an inherently hostile field, peopled by "older White males, who were unsympathetic, uncaring, and unavailable," revealed a 2002 study of African-Americans' attitudes toward psychotherapy and psychotherapists. "Psychologists were perceived as predisposed to viewing African Americans as 'crazy' and prone to labeling strong expressions of emotion as illness."Black patients, the authors found, came to these encounters fearing being misdiagnosed, labeled, and brainwashed. "A common characterization was that psychologists were 'impersonal.' Psychologists were described as elitist and too far removed from the community to be of assistance to most African Americans."

There is undoubtedly a fair amount of truth behind the perception that mental health specialists are too removed to relate to minority children, particularly when it comes to the care of children with mental health issues in the inner city. For there are some unique barriers—attitudinal as well as logistical—standing in the way of bringing the best possible mental health care to poorer children. There are a lot of urban myths circulating in less-affluent, less-educated communities about the causes of psychiatric disorders and about psychotropic medication. Employers won't give workers time off to attend school conferences or medical appointments, and teachers, focused on training their students to do well on standardized tests, won't take time out of their lesson plans to work on behavioral management.

Doctors aren't necessarily tuned-in or sympathetic to any of this. In fact, a number of those quoted in a 2005 study said they simply didn't want to treat inner-city minority children with mental health issues, because they found the job too challenging. "I can't offer [parents] the time that they need to discuss the problems," one doctor said. "I can't offer them behavior therapy, and they need that." Doctors and school staff also told the study's authors that inner-city parents were too "disorganized, misinformed, and inconsistent" to aid in their children's care. One pediatrician said that the protocols for dealing with ADHD in particular were written with "highly organized" middle- and upper-income families in mind and couldn't be put in action with a poorer population.

"The finger-pointing bred distrust," the study's authors dryly concluded.

The North Carolina mother, a human-resources manager, had to brace herself, time and again, against just this sort of insult of low expectations, as she fought the school system to advocate for her son. "I was very afraid of letting schools know he had [depression]. I just figured they would categorize him and that would be the end of it, so I had to stay *very* involved," she told me. "The school personnel was surprised I was so engaged. A lot of that was racial: That wasn't their experience with black parents."

But, like the mothers in Texas and D.C. I mentioned earlier, this mother had one distinct advantage: she had the personal resources and the wherewithal to *fight.* "I'm a salaried employee," she told me. "How do you do it if you have an hourly wage?"

Children with severe mental illness and their families have the greatest needs—and are right now faring the worst in our current system of non-care. Over the past two decades, insurance companies have stopped paying for long-term inpatient care for mentally ill children. As a result, psychiatric hospitals have been steadily closing, and residential treatment programs for the most difficult children, where tuition is most often paid with public funds, are packed.

Ideally, experts say, even chronically and severely mentally ill children should be cared for at home, with wraparound services provided within their communities. They should have things like therapeutic afterschool, community-based outpatient services, and short-term transitional residential care centers. In general, none of this exists. Instead, if children become dangerously manic, or suicidally depressed, or psychotic, they end up in emergency rooms, where there's often no child psychiatrist to see them. If they're admitted to a hospital, they generally end up on adult psych wards that at worst can be terrifying, and at best simply aren't adapted to meet their needs.

The result of all this fractured, fragmented, chaotic, or nonexistent care, according to Christopher Bellonci, a psychiatrist who is the medical director of the Walker School, a nonprofit residential treatment program in Needham, Massachusetts, is that children with psychiatric problems get steadily worse, and eventually "fail up" through repeated trials of medication and short-term hospitalizations until they can no longer be kept at home. "Some of these kids end up at higher levels of care because their issues are not addressed early enough," Bellonci told me.

Many who reach this level of need are victims of abuse and neglect. Many have parents who themselves are mentally ill and can't properly care for their children. Many others have parents who are simply desperate. Because of the paucity of resources, because of the enormous cost of getting care for the sickest kids, and because of private insurance's refusal now to pay for extended hospital or residential treatment stays, some loving, capable parents are actually now forced to make their children wards of the state in order to get the child-welfare system to pay for their care. In Virginia, in 2004, one in four children in the foster-care system were there either because their parents were desperate to find for them mental health services that their insurance fully covered or because their parents did not have access to any insurance at all.

"Parents who have not been abusive or neglectful are put in the untenable situation of having to surrender custody," Bellonci said. "It's criminal, frankly."

The most dramatic illustration of this impossible situation came in

2008 when thirty-six children were abandoned in Nebraska after the state adopted a "Safe Haven" law permitting parents to drop off their kids at designated locations and hand their care over to state authorities without risk of legal recourse. Most of the abandoned kids had serious mental health issues. Thirty had previously received mental health care, and eleven had formerly been in residential care. Some of the kids had been on waiting lists for months for spots in residential treatment programs. Seven of them had come from out of state, including one who'd been driven 1,000 miles to Lincoln, Nebraska, from Smyrna, Georgia.

As the crisis escalated, one Oklahoma woman who had been struggling to get her adopted foster child into a residential treatment program called a Nebraska official and threatened to bring her son to his state unless she was helped quickly. Calls were made, and the boy was admitted to a local psychiatric program within days.

"Why on God's green earth does it take all that to get help?" the mother asked the *Omaha World-Herald.*

Why indeed?

Why, for that matter, at a moment in time when help—good help—exists for kids with all kinds of mental health issues, are we as a society so caught up in debating the reality of those issues, second-guessing parents, blaming sick kids for being "bad," conducting, in short, an eternal, national referendum on the state of Science and Society, instead of trying to make things better for children and their families?

Why is there so little empathy for children with mental health issues and, in particular, their parents? Why is there so much sniping, so much suspicion and doubt and skepticism, so much stigma, generally? Why, in particular, has parent-blaming remained so pervasive and so pernicious, so far outlasting the prior prejudices of mental health professionals?

This whole poisonous web of belief and disbelief has less to do, I believe, with real parents, real children, and their real issues than it does with larger issues people have right now in our society. It has to do with all the ways in which people have come to feel they are besieged and that their children are particularly vulnerable. It has to do with the fact that the biggest fault line dividing parents these days is competition for resources, which results in the pervasive feeling that other people are unfairly pushing their children forward and that one's own children are, or may soon be, as one suburban Maryland mom once put it to me, "left behind in the dust."

Fear about our children's performance, about their future, about their ability to survive and thrive in an increasingly callous and competitive world, is the dominant theme of parenthood today. That, I believe, is the main reason the myths and stereotypes about parents who medicate or otherwise seek mental health care or accommodations for their children have gotten so much traction.

Most people don't like to face head-on the sense that their own families are at a disadvantage. They don't like to admit to jealousy, fear, and resentment—even to themselves. And so, I believe, they displace those negative feelings onto others. Some of the most pointed hostility I have heard toward parents whose children take medication or engage in other nondrug therapies for problems that to outsiders seem to have questionable validity reeks of this particular form of fear and jealousy and competition.

It is, after all, so much easier to scapegoat a group that is already vulnerable and socially stigmatized—parents of children with mental health issues—than to face one's own worries, and insecurities, and fears. In other words, our issues are getting in the way of our clearly seeing, and being able to help, kids with issues.

· 6 ·

"B-a-d" Children, Worse Parents (and Even Worse Doctors)

When it comes to the popular idea that vast numbers of normal kids are being pathologized, therapized, and stuffed full of meds by careless doctors and lazy parents, the facts just aren't there.

So why do so many people persist in believing the overdrugged and overdiagnosed child story line?

Well, for one thing, it's easy to think the worst these days of doctors—particularly the psychiatric-drug-prescribing kind. The many stories that have made their way into the news over the past few years about psychiatrists' enmeshment with the pharmaceutical industry have been damning. Given what we've learned about drugmakers' payments to psychiatrists, control of published research, and financial ties to government regulators, it's not unreasonable to approach the matter of giving kids psychotropic medications with distrust and suspicion. (I'll go into more detail about all of that a bit later.)

But first—what of the equally strong distrust and suspicion of parents that's expressed by the "naysayer" view? How is it that there's such a sense that many parents are looking for a "quick fix" way to shut up and control their less-than-adorable kids?

The truth is, it isn't just a reasoned wariness of psychiatrists that inspires and sustains that Overmedicated Child story line. Many people also think pretty badly of today's parents, too. And, for that matter, of today's children.

Kids these days, you hear all the time, are badly behaved, atrociously ill-mannered. They're narcissistic, entitled, out of control. The "rudest in history," as an MSNBC headline unflinchingly put it, in 2009.

These are children so unsocialized that only 9 percent of respondents, according to surveys done by the public opinion research group Public Agenda earlier this decade, were able to say that the kids they saw in public were "respectful toward adults." Toddlers so emotionally unself-regulated that they are being expelled from preschool. Schoolchildren so undisciplined that, even in kindergarten, they use expletives with teachers, and bite, kick, and hit other children.

In 2004, more than one in three teachers told pollsters they had seriously considered leaving their profession or knew a colleague who had left because of "intolerable" student behavior. *Time* magazine, in a much-noted story called "Does Kindergarten Need Cops?" told of an alarming rise in explosive and aggressive behavior in young children nationwide, and quoted a woman who worked with emotionally disturbed children in the Fort Worth Independent School District's Psychological Services department to say that out-of-control behavior wasn't just a special-ed issue in the public schools anymore; it was a new kind of normal.

"We have our ED kids," the educator said, "and then we have our b-a-d kids."

Dissecting and chronicling how "b-a-d" today's children really are has become something of a national pastime. A Chicago café owner made headlines far beyond his city when he handed out an open letter that spoke of an "epidemic" of antisocial behavior among his youngest patrons, and was rewarded with a boycott by angry local parents. The preschool expulsions, too, sparked a gleeful round of social commentary.

Particularly fired up on the "b-a-d" child topic were social commentators on the right, like John Rosemond, the syndicated columnist and family psychologist who has regaled readers with tales of "disruptive urchins" who "obviously have yet to have been taught the basic rudiments of public behavior," and do things like roller-skate around tables or watch DVDs at four-star restaurants.

But children—as the angry Chicago parents (bashed by the café owner in *The New York Times* as "former cheerleaders and beauty queens" who "have a very strong sense of entitlement") knew—have not truly been the objects of the vitriol and condemnation that have accompanied accounts of bad kid behavior. The real targets are mothers and fathers. The current generation of parents—working parents, baby-boomer parents, and "Gen X" parents who espouse the "attachment"-enhancing views of the baby-wearing, cosleeping, long-term-breast-feeding guru Dr. William Sears—are now being singled out for blame for a whole host of children's problems.

Too much self-esteem building, too much focus on children's emotional well-being, too much "attachment" to parents generally, and not enough concern for others, onlookers and experts typically say, have made children self-centered, arrogant, and narcissistic. Too much money, too much stuff, too much indulgence, and too little self-reliance and exposure to boredom, is resulting in kids who are insatiable in their needs for novelty and distraction, plagued by dissatisfaction, and incapable of tolerating frustration or aloneness.

Today's parents, we read over and over, and saw for a time in shows like *Nanny 911* and *Supernanny*, are incompetent. They can't say no. They have no patience. They have no manners themselves. They outsource etiquette lessons to special schools run by proper-seeming matrons (or did, in the money-flush years leading up to the Great Recession). They call up parent coaches for help with discipline. They meet with experts who can script them on how to stand strong in the face of demands for new iPods, cell phones, Game Boys, clothes, and cars.

They're simply useless. And, many people now believe, these hapless parents avoid taking responsibility for their witless deeds by blaming any problems that arise at home on their children. A respondent to my column on the "Ritalin Wars" put it perfectly: "I look around and I see almost no stay-at-home parents amongst our circle of acquaintances and I wonder how well these parents understand their children with such limited exposure to them and I wonder if they are feeling guilty about being unable to spend time with them," he wrote. "So my thesis is that parents' guilt about not being around their kids combined with their discomfort with kids' behavior may result in compensating by eagerly digesting the latest kids' malady du jour and perhaps going so far as to seek treatment for their own kids. What else can they do to feel like they're helping their kids?"

The problem with parents, we were told, went far beyond incompetence, though. When it came to b-a-d behavior, many parents were worse than their kids. They attacked each other at soccer games. They screamed at—even physically assaulted—coaches who made calls that disadvantaged their kids. They leaned on teachers and even college professors for better grades for their children. They refused to make their kids take responsibility for poor grades or their own bad behavior, marginalizing teachers so thoroughly that, by 2004, more than half of educators surveyed said they ended up being soft on discipline because they couldn't count on parents or schools to support them. "Parents are the new class of bullies," the *Milwaukee Journal Sentinel* declared in 2006.

What all this came down to, at base, was a warped sense of child advocacy. With competition for resources getting fiercer, and the road to success getting narrower, many parents feel it's their duty to make sure their children aren't left behind—ever. Behind the bullying, behind the obnoxious behavior, this basic worry screams: Will my child make it? Will he or she have what it takes to survive?

Some parents, crippled by insecurity and lacking faith in their kids, are willing to resort to outright cheating to make sure their kids will thrive. They hold their boys back in school for a year to make sure they'll have a leg up academically, socially, and in sports. (Some, it must be said, are pushed into doing this by schools, which have so beefed up their kindergarten curriculum that some boys—it's usually boys—just can't hack it.)

Some resort to much more sinister forms of stature-boosting, like giving kids growth hormone to make sure they'll be able to stand tall among their peers. In 2008 it was reported that some 40 percent of children currently being given growth hormone to increase their height didn't actually have an inherent growth-hormone deficiency or other genetic disorder that was adversely affecting their growth. They were just short, and their parents didn't want them to be.

I think it's fair to assume that parents who go to lengths such as these are rare. But the actions of those who do things like cheat their genes have had a disproportionate impact on the national psyche at a time when everyone is already convinced that everyone else is (more successfully) jockeying for advantage. Thus, Michael J. Sandel, a professor of political philosophy at Harvard, writing on the growing use of non-medically necessary growth hormone in children in the *Atlantic* in 2004, worried that this practice could be "collectively self-defeating" for our nation's youth. "As some become taller, others become shorter relative to the norm," he wrote. "As the unenhanced began to feel shorter, they, too, might seek treatment, leading to a hormonal arms race that left everyone worse off; especially those who couldn't afford to buy their way up from shortness."

Outrageous as that particular thought might seem, there were indications, as the decade advanced, that children themselves were engaging in similar sorts of races for unfair advantage, and not so rarely at that. In 2005 came reports that girls as young as age nine were using steroids to boost their academic performance—and give themselves a more sculpted look to boot. Another study in *Pediatrics* showed one in eight boys and one in twelve girls saying they used either hormones or supplements to improve their appearance, muscle mass, or strength.

And plain old academic cheating was epidemic. Gary Pavella, director of judicial programs and student ethical development for the University of Maryland, College Park, informed a journalism conference I attended a few years ago that a "culture of academic dishonesty" reigns now on college campuses, engaging fully one-third of students at many universities. In the fall of 2008, as what was being billed as the most competitive college admissions season in history kicked off, *The New York Times* reported that more than 90 percent of high school students said they'd cheated in one way or another. And the *Chicago Tribune* revealed that students applying to college had begun artfully sabotaging their competitors' efforts, sending anonymous letters to college admissions officers to report on rivals' alcohol use, Facebook follies, or . . . cheating. "Nothing shocks us anymore," said Christopher Watson, dean of undergraduate admission at Northwestern University.

In this climate, it's easy to see why people would view parents' efforts to secure special-education services for their kids as a cynical play for unfair advantage. And why they would view disorders like ADHD—even dyslexia—essentially as cooked-up excuses for children's bad behavior, parents' lack of competency, and society's refusal to acknowledge that some kids just can't compete as well as others.

As I noted earlier, some commentators and financially interested parties (like school districts being sued by parents) have managed, in recent years, to cast serious doubt on the reality of many children's learning disabilities. The same lacerating doubt has continually been aired, over the course of the past decade, at children with other mental health issues, most notably ADHD.

Given the way people feel about children, it's very easy to paint ADHD as a kind of conduct disorder, chiefly characterized by b-a-d behavior—a sign of "toddlerhood in perpetuity," as John Rosemond and his coauthor Bose Ravenel described it (and oppositional defiant disorder and early-onset bipolar disorder) in their 2008 book, *The Diseasing of America's Children.* For years, the ADHD child has been painted as a wiggly, badly behaved boy who's been giving his parents and teachers hell and needs nothing more than the modern-day equivalent of a good kick in the pants. This child is highly amenable to behavior-modification techniques, doesn't have any of the cognitive deficits considered by experts to be the core elements of ADHD (those not so therapy-tractable things like poor working memory), and is highly likely to outgrow his symptoms as he ages. In short, he (for it's always a "he") is just a bad—kind of immature, kind of normal—boy.

Given the way people feel about parents, it's been even easier to paint psychotropic drug use—and stimulant use for ADHD in particular—as an effort by parents to "improve their children," as a 2003 report from the Bush White House, shocking in its degree of disdain and disrespect for the country's mothers and fathers, put it. The report, *Beyond Therapy: Biotechnology and the Pursuit of Happiness,* compiled by the President's Council on Bioethics, contained a large section dedicated to the topic of the "pursuit of better-behaved and more competent children through the use of drugs."

"The growing availability of a wide range of behavior-modifying drugs," the authors wrote:

> *". . . will invite many parents at least to consider their use, in order to realize more effectively various aspirations they have for their children. And if other people's children are already using them for similar purposes, many parents may feel pressed to give them a try, in order not to deny to their own child an opportunity for greater success. Competitive behavior of many parents seeking advantages for their children is already*

widespread in schooling and sports programs; there is no reason to believe that it will stop at the border of psychotropic drugs, should they prove effective and safe."

The authors offered no evidence that parents were actually using stimulants to create "better children." But it was clear that, in their opinion, if such "enhancement" was not already happening, it soon would be. "Ritalin and similar stimulants," they wrote, "can be, and quite possibly are being, used to mollify or improve children who suffer no disorder except childhood and childishness."

One could sense this view of parents running through much of the reporting on children's mental health issues in the past few years. *Frontline*'s highly disturbing 2008 documentary on "the medicated child," for example, showed bipolar children taking dizzying numbers of drugs, their stories intercut with references to four-year-old Rebecca Riley from Hull, Massachusetts, who died in 2006 after her parents gave her an overdose of similar meds, without any evidence that the children featured might really need them. You saw, for example, extremely upsetting footage of a teenage boy named Jacob, who had at one time been put on eight medications simultaneously, and was left with a terrible, neck-wrenching tic, without ever seeing or hearing what sorts of extreme behaviors had led his parents to agree to such extreme measures in the first place. The mother of a heavily medicated four-year-old boy said his need for drugs was "do or die," yet his angel face made her words sound like a lie.

"Don't you think she'll grow out of it?" *Frontline*'s reporter at one point needled the mother of a quite reasonable, if sad-looking, bipolar twelve-year-old who at five had gleefully fantasized about decapitating her parents.

"No," the mother had answered, in tears. "She'll have to take medications for the rest of her life if she wants to go to college or have a job or have a family."

Since the kids just didn't seem sick, the parents' self-justifications rang suspiciously hollow.

News reporting on ADHD medication use has similarly and consistently cast doubt upon both the appropriateness of stimulant use and the seriousness of the ADHD diagnosis. Time and again, ADHD meds have been presented as nothing more than a cheating aid—"the steroids of intellect," to borrow a phrase from the headline of a column that ran in the University of Connecticut's *The Daily Campus* in 2004. The drugs were an SAT score-booster in *The Wall Street Journal* and a homework-helper for crazed overachievers in the weekly *Washingtonian* magazine, which in 2006 devoted a long feature to supercompetitive local kids and college students trying to up their grades and test scores by abusing ADHD meds.

"In the 1960s, the Rolling Stones dubbed tranquilizers and antidepressants 'mother's little helper.' Forty years later, Adderall is 'brother's little helper,'" *Washingtonian* writer Harry Jaffe reported. "Prescribed liberally by psychiatrists to young people who they believe have a learning disability," he noted, Adderall, in "street terms" is "'speed' in a very low dose."

Jaffe's "believe" said it all; the stimulants weren't being used to address problems that were real, they weren't being used to help impaired children and teens level the playing field with their peers—to "be like everyone else," as an eleven-year-old on Concerta once put it to me—but as a means to *out*perform all others. On the *Washingtonian*'s website, Jaffe's piece was accompanied by a teaser for a thematically related article, "Can You Get Me In?" about the practice of paying consultants to help toddlers gain access to top private schools. The message of the juxtaposition: The wealthy are doing everything in their power to get ahead of you—through money, through connections, through pills.

The abuse of stimulants—admittedly now rife in competitive high schools and on college campuses—and the proper use of the drugs have been conflated in media coverage. In a 2006 story, "Can You Find Concentration in a Bottle?" *Time* magazine repeatedly referred to Ritalin as a "popular performance aid." In 2007, once the news spread that even *professors* were using pills like the mind-sharpener Modafinil to boost their academic output, the anxiety that parents might be using drugs like Ritalin or Adderall to give their kids a leg up over others metastasized. The *Los Angeles Times* ("They're Bulking Up Mentally") proposed that drugs should perhaps be banned for anyone—with or without attention deficit—taking the SAT. A bioethicist from the University of Pennsylvania said that "she was beginning to detect resentment toward students who used the drugs from classmates who did not" and "wondered whether improving productivity through artificial means also might undermine the value of hard work."

The tragedy and cruelty of all this is that kids with ADHD are now doubly burdened: first, with their disorder (and with the not-very-welcome need to take medication) and then with the stigma of being perceived as cheaters. The effect of this stigma is something no one engaged in all the fretting about "enhancement," "authenticity," and good old-fashioned human values has seemed much concerned with. It has hurt children, of course. It has ruffled feathers among parents. It has been a major irritant to doctors seeking to improve knowledge about and the treatment of ADHD and other disorders. But in the course of this particular debate, those particular doctors have rarely been given anything other than parenthetical space in which to air their views.

After all, children and parents aren't the only people about whom Americans are predisposed to think the very worst these days. Many also have an atrociously low opinion of psychiatrists.

In part, it's for good reason. The past few years have brought a spate of truly stomach-turning revelations about the degree to which some prominent psychiatrists, including very prominent child psychiatrists, have been in bed with the pharmaceutical industry.

In May 2007, *The New York Times* ran an exposé based upon an analysis of records in Minnesota, which showed that, between 1997 and 2005, more than a third of the state's licensed psychiatrists took money from drug companies. The median payment to psychiatrists was $1,750, though one was paid more than $689,000 by drugmakers from 1998 to 2004, doing so many paid lectures that, she told the *Times*, "it was hard for me to find time to see patients in my clinical practice." Another psychiatrist, a clinician and researcher at the University of Minnesota, said the thousands of dollars he earned giving marketing lectures for Johnson & Johnson were an important supplement to his income.

"Academics don't get paid very much," said the doctor, whose university salary was $196,310. "If I was an entertainer, I think I would certainly do a lot better."

Dr. Melissa DelBello, a psychiatrist at the University of Cincinnati, was singled out by the *Times* for her work promoting the use of atypical antipsychotics to treat children with bipolar disorder. She had led a study that claimed good results for the antipsychotic Seroquel, made by AstraZeneca, in treating bipolar teenagers, even though so many of those teens dropped out of the study that in the end, it comprised a sample size of only eight. AstraZeneca then hired Dr. DelBello, who was earning $183,500 as a professor, to give sponsored talks.

"Trust me, I don't make much," she told the *Times*, when asked about the price of her consulting for the drug company.

That quotation caught the eye of Senator Charles Grassley of Iowa. He decided to follow up and see just how much that "not much" was. Grassley, since 2004, had been following what he viewed as the "too cozy relationship" between the Food and Drug Administration and Big Pharma; now he turned his sights on the relationships between drugmakers and doctors. From University of Cincinnati disclosure forms, he discovered that Dr. DelBello had claimed about $100,000 in outside income from 2005 to 2007. AstraZeneca told his office, however, that it had paid her more than $238,000 in that period.

Grassley's investigations intensified. In June, 2008, his office revealed that Dr. Joseph Biederman, the controversial child psychiatrist at Harvard Medical School, had earned at least $1.6 million from pharmaceutical companies between 2000 and 2007, while reporting only several hundred thousand dollars in outside income to university authorities. Other child psychiatrists at Harvard were implicated, too.

In June of 2008, Grassley also raised questions about Dr. Alan F. Schatzberg of Stanford, then the incoming president of the American Psychiatric Association, whose $4.8 million stock holdings in a drug development company raised conflict-of-interest concerns for the senator. Grassley requested that the American Psychiatric Association—which in 2006 had received 30 percent of its $62.5 million in financing from the pharmaceutical industry—provide a complete accounting of all of its revenues from pharmaceutical companies since 2003. And he followed up with the revelation that Dr. Charles B. Nemeroff, a well-known psychiatrist at Emory University, had failed to report at least $1.2 million of his more than $2.8 million income from consulting for drug companies between 2000 and 2008. In late 2008, Nemeroff voluntarily gave up his post as department chair and said, "I regret the failure of full disclosure on my part. . . . I believe that I was acting in good faith to comply with the rules as I understood them." In addition, Emory said it would not submit any NIH or other sponsored grant in which Nemeroff was listed as an investigator or had any other role for a period of two years.

After this long round of public humiliation and comeuppance, psychiatrists began to push back. DelBello eventually complained that she had been misquoted by the *Times*, saying her comment that she did not "make much" from drug companies had come in response to a reporter's question "about how much money she was given for making a single, individual presentation." Schatzberg told *The New York Times* he had "fully complied" with Stanford's disclosure policies and federal guidelines regarding his research, and Stanford University vigorously protested the accusations made against him. And the American Psychiatric Association objected that psychiatrists in general were being unfairly singled out for notice.

The APA had a point—but only up to a point.

The practice of drug and device makers enlisting doctors to serve as part of their marketing corps—as paid lecturers, for example, or by putting their names on research papers ghostwritten by industry flacks—isn't limited to psychiatry. Neither is the practice of consulting for drugmakers, serving on their corporate boards, or having other financial stakes in the pharmaceutical industry.

Conflicts of interest between the pharmaceutical industry and prominent research physicians "permeate the clinical research enterprise," wrote Dr. Marcia Angell, author of the 2004 *The Truth About the Drug Companies* and the former editor in chief of *The New England Journal of Medicine*, in *The Journal of the American Medical Association* in 2008. About two-thirds of academic medical centers have financial stakes in companies that sponsor research within their facilities, her research found; two-thirds of medical school department chairs receive departmental income, and three-fifths receive personal income, from drug companies.

Doctors are prohibited by law from accepting drug company payment for prescribing particular drugs. But they can pad their income with speaking and consulting fees, and they can accept expensive meals and trips from drugmakers, if such pleasures are encountered in the pursuit of the "continuing medical education" that they're required to do in order to stay current in their field. Continuing medical education is increasingly provided and paid for by the pharmaceutical industry. In 2008, half of all continuing medical education in the United States was funded by drug companies.

Medical education in general was increasingly being underwritten by drug funds, too, as drug companies lost no time in teaching cash-poor medical students just where their bread was buttered. Ninety-seven percent of third-year medical students in 2008 went out to dinner with a drug rep. Ninety percent of those students received drugmaker gifts, according to Eric Campbell, an associate professor of medicine at Harvard University and researcher with Massachusetts General Hospital's Institute for Health Policy. "They start these kids in medical school; all they're doing is training them to take stuff," he told me.

"The drug companies own medicine in America," said Campbell, who studies the relationship between academia and industry. "They own research, education, and patient care. Relationships between doctors and drug companies, researchers and institutions involved in medical care and drug companies, are ubiquitous. At the individual level, specialists are more likely to have these relationships than nonspecialists," he noted. But, he added, "to the best I can tell, the frequency of relationships with industry are very similar across all fields."

Grassley's investigations did not, in fact, focus uniquely upon psychiatrists. Cardiologists, for example, also came in for considerable scrutiny, as did orthopedic surgeons, and the amounts of money or the value of the trips and meals these specialists received often far exceeded typical payments to psychiatrists. Indeed, the stories that emerged on conflicts of interest between the orthopedic surgeons and, in particular, the device maker Medtronic, detailed in *The Wall Street Journal* in 2008, were far more eye-catching than the psychiatrist stories, as they involved trips to Alaska, Orlando, and Las Vegas, as well as "VIP visits" to a Memphis strip club named Platinum Plus.

But the idea of psychiatry as a force of corruption has a particular hold on the American imagination, and it was the psychiatrists under investigation by Grassley who got the lion's share of media attention. The Biederman case was such good drama that a fictional version of it even made its way onto an episode of *Boston Legal*, where Candice Bergen's character, Shirley Schmidt, railed to a jury, "A famed Harvard psychiatrist helped fuel the recent boom in antipsychotics for kids. Turns out he personally took over $1.6 million from drugmakers over the past seven years. He also failed to report this income to the university, by the way. How can this be?"

The Biederman revelations had a particular vindicating quality for all those who'd long felt that there was something rotten in the state of children's mental health care. Biederman was, after all, the Massachusetts General Hospital doctor who'd pioneered and popularized the adult bipolar diagnosis in children. He'd aggressively promoted the use of powerful new "atypical" antipsychotics and mood stabilizers in very young children. His research had long been criticized for its small sample sizes, its symptom criteria, and the extreme youth of its subjects. And the atypical antipsychotics really were worrisome.

They'd been sold to psychiatrists as a great improvement over older antipsychotics, like Thorazine or Haldol, which had been used (in hospital settings) in prior decades to calm the kind of out-of-control children who were now being labeled "bipolar." The older drugs (often called "major tranquilizers") were known to cause very serious neurological side effects that made kids stiff or shaky, or left them riddled with tics or other abnormal involuntary movements. The new drugs were said to be much less likely to cause these side effects. But they turned out to have serious side effects of their own: notably, metabolic changes that could lead to enormous and rapid weight gain, heart and pulmonary problems, high blood sugar, blood lipid changes, and diabetes.

Although only Risperdal was approved for use in kids (and this not until 2007), the atypical antipsychotics were, thanks to the research and "education" efforts of some doctors, frequently prescribed "off-label" to children in the decade following their introduction to the market in the 1990s. There was virtually no research to support this vastly expanding use. By 2008, a number of states were suing the atypicals' makers for inappropriately promoting their off-label use in children, among other groups. Many prominent psychiatrists, including ones who believed that there were appropriate uses for the atypical antipsychotics in some children, were raising the alarm about overprescription and about the dangers of the drugs which, critics charged, had been criminally downplayed by the drugmakers. These dangers were not inconsequential. FDA data collected from 2000 to 2004 showed at least forty-five deaths of children in which an atypical antipsychotic was listed as the "primary suspect," and, in 2006, antipsychotics were listed in FDA reports as the "primary suspect" in the deaths of at least twenty-nine children and serious side effects in at least 165 more. (And as adverse-effect reporting to the FDA is voluntary, the agency's lists of drug-related deaths and side effects are generally considered to represent a tiny fraction of those that actually occur.)

The revelations about Harvard's Joseph Biederman appeared to confirm the claims of child psychiatry's worst critics: The man who'd mainstreamed the use of atypical antipsychotics in children really was in the pocket of the drug companies. The whole practice of medicating kids early and aggressively—a practice Biederman was largely credited with having pioneered—could, in this case at least, be attributed pretty convincingly to the machinations of the "medicopharmaceutical industrial complex."

As time passed, the Biederman news only got worse. In November 2008, e-mails emerged between Johnson & Johnson, the manufacturer of Risperdal, and Biederman, showing that the doctor had pressured the company to fund a research center that he would head at Massachusetts General Hospital with the expressed purpose of attempting to "move forward the commercial goals of J&J." By the end of the year, Mass General had launched a formal investigation of Biederman's apparent conflicts of interest. In a letter to *The Boston Globe* in December 2008,

Biederman defended himself against conflict-of-interest charges, writing, "Any implications that J&J's interest interfered with the Center's work is wrong. Indeed, I have published research critical of J&J compounds. I never owned J&J stock; and whether the company succeeded financially had no importance to me." Nonetheless, the doctor agreed to stop all work paid for by the drug companies and removed himself from industry-financed research at the hospital.

How many other psychiatrists are in the pay of Big Pharma—and to what extent—is impossible to know as of this writing. Minnesota, Vermont, Maine, and West Virginia are the only states to require some kind of public disclosure of industry payments to doctors. The very partial information they provide has created a damning portrait so far. When the state of Vermont released a report on pharmaceutical marketing disclosures in July 2008, it found that psychiatrists were overrepresented among the state's top one hundred recipients of drug money, with eleven psychiatrists alone receiving approximately 20 percent of the total value of drug payments to the state's doctors. When *The New York Times*, in May 2007, analyzed records of drugmaker payments to Minnesota psychiatrists, it found an extremely problematic link between doctors' payments and their prescribing patterns.

From 2000 to 2005, the *Times* revealed, payments to the psychiatrists rose more than sixfold, while prescriptions of antipsychotics for children in the state's Medicaid program rose more than ninefold. "Those who took the most money from makers of atypicals tended to prescribe the drugs to children the most often, the data suggest," wrote reporters Gardiner Harris, Benedict Carey, and Janet Roberts. "On average, Minnesota psychiatrists who received at least $5,000 from atypical makers from 2000 to 2005 appear to have written three times as many atypical prescriptions for children as psychiatrists who received less or no money."

Most prominent academic journals now require authors to list their industry affiliations at the end of their articles. This is a salutary development, but the revelations can be disheartening. To take just one example:

In 2007, the long-awaited three-year follow-up to the *Multimodal Treatment Study of Children with Attention Deficit Hyperactivity Disorder* was published, and listed at the end all the outside links its participants had had to drug companies since the study had begun in 1992. The MTA study, as it's called, is the most comprehensive comparative study of ADHD treatments ever conducted. It is entirely funded by the federal government, with no drug-industry money. And yet, all of the psychiatrists had at some point had at least one relationship with a drugmaker, and most had had several. Half the psychologists, for that matter, did, too.

The MTA researchers are among the leading lights in their field. Their work is of vital importance for helping doctors and parents make decisions about how to treat ADHD. There's no indication that industry ties influenced their findings. But their industry affiliations (past or present) make them easy, indeed unavoidable, targets for the cynicism and doubt of those who believe that the use of psychotropic medication by kids is a big drug industry–funded plot.

I happen to believe in the basic soundness of the psychiatric enterprise; that mental disorders are real, are at least in part biological in origin, can cause as much suffering as other medical disorders, can have a high fatality rate, and can be helped, at least in part, by medication. The psychiatric researchers and practitioners I interviewed for this book struck me as genuinely motivated by a desire to help children, and genuinely concerned about the effects of drug-company money on prescribing and research (though many argued there wouldn't be much research without it). I see the pollution of psychiatry by drug money as a tragedy, a wasted opportunity, a very self-destructive move for a profession that needs to gain the public trust in order to work for the public good.

Being joined at the hip with the pharmaceutical industry is just about the worst possible way to move toward earning that trust. For the industry, time and again, has shamed itself through its commercial practices, manipulating data to make drugs look more effective than they are, suppressing information about bad, even fatal, side effects, bringing new drugs to market that are no more effective than older and cheaper ones, and encouraging physicians to prescribe drugs to patients for whom they're unnecessary and even dangerous.

The industry's behavior has colored Americans' perceptions of psychiatry to the point that, in many people's minds, there's no actual difference between the practices of psychiatrists and the machinations of drug marketers. This is, I believe, an unjustified perception. And yet, as with most overblown public perceptions, it contains a kernel of truth.

The pharmaceutical industry now has an outsized influence over the practice of both child and adult psychiatry, and not only because of direct cash payments to doctors, universities, or the APA. It also has a greatly disproportionate power to control the very knowledge base upon which doctors—whether in the pay of Big Pharma or not—make patient care decisions. And it has not been using that power judiciously.

The pharmaceutical and biotech industries fund the lion's share of clinical trials of new drugs in our country—60 percent of those clinical studies in 2004. This wasn't always the case with research into children's psychiatric medications. In the 1980s and early 1990s, what studies there were on the use of psychotropic drugs in children—on the use of stimulants, tricyclic antidepressants, and SSRIs—came from the National Institute of Mental Health, and there simply wasn't much commercial interest in testing drugs on children, particularly when doctors were willing to simply prescribe adult drugs to them off-label.

It was partly to try to put some limits on that off-label prescribing and partly to get more information on how drugs specifically affected kids, that lawmakers in 1997 offered the pharmaceutical industry a sweetened deal: If drugmakers would run pediatric research trials with their new products, they could have six months of additional patent protection when their new drugs went to market. While this legislation, the FDA Modernization Act of 1997, has somewhat increased the available information on how medications affect children—about a third of the drugs used in children now have pediatric prescribing information on the product label—the government's financial incentive hasn't produced anything like the vast increase in reliable information for child psychiatrists, pediatricians, and parents that it was intended to create.

There's far too little information still, and because doctors continue to prescribe adult drugs to kids off-label, it can trickle down to office practice far too late. Yet it isn't just the quantity of information that's lacking; the quality of information that has emerged in the era of industry-sponsored research has been sorely deficient, too.

For one thing, the pharmaceutical industry only funds studies on drugs it can make money with—new drugs that companies want to bring to market—and doesn't test older drugs or set up comparisons between new drugs and older ones. For another, the industry doesn't spend much on the studies that seek to find out if its drugs cause any harm once they've gone to market.

There are other considerable downsides to having the pharmaceutical industry run its own show in terms of running drug trials: the data collected during drug trials paid for by pharmaceutical companies generally belongs to those companies, and the company can decide when or whether to publish its results. Negative studies don't necessarily make it into the public eye. (This was shown most grotesquely in 2004, when the news broke that drug giant SmithKline Beecham—later GlaxoSmithKline—had decided in 1998 to suppress clinical trial data that, as an internal company memo put it, were "commercially unacceptable," and would "undermine the profile of paroxetine," or its soon-to-be blockbuster Paxil. The company published a study saying that Paxil was "generally well tolerated and effective formajor depression in adolescents" even though two clinical trials had shown the drug to be no more—and sometimes less—effective in fighting depression than a placebo, and five times more likely to cause extreme emotionality or suicidal thoughts or behavior. As noted earlier, this resulted in a lawsuit by New York State and the company's ultimately publishing all test results.)

The result of all this, a report on "Child and Adolescent Psychopharmacology in the New Millennium" in the *Journal of the American Academy of Child & Adolescent Psychiatry*, stated, in 2006, is that there is "little or no randomized evidence on which to base clinical practice" in using psychotropic drugs on children. The more than decade-old government incentives to drugmakers to test drugs in children, it seems, have brought virtually no payoff for prescribing doctors and concerned families. "Drugs are often widely prescribed to youth, without evidence of safety or efficacy from controlled studies," the 2006 *JAACAP* report concluded.

As I write this, the state legal actions against Big Pharma (brought by states after investigations showed large numbers of patients being treated with off-label medications, something Medicaid policy normally does not permit), just keep coming. In late 2007, a number of state attorneys general began suing the makers of atypical antipsychotics, charging the drugmakers were illegally promoting their use for "non-medically necessary uses," as Arkansas Attorney General Dustin McDaniel stated in his suit against Johnson & Johnson and its Janssen units. Janssen alone was accused, by nine state attorneys general, of having urged doctors to prescribe the atypical antipsychotic Risperdal for a host of non-FDA-approved uses in treating conditions like depression and anxiety disorders, and even ADHD. In fact, although Risperdal, experts say, has no role whatsoever in treating ADHD (except, perhaps, as a kind of elephant tranquilizer for kids with severe behavioral problems who also happen to carry an ADHD diagnosis), a federal regulatory panel found in the fall of 2008 that fully 16 percent of the pediatric users of the medication were taking it for that purpose.

In early 2009, the United States Justice Department charged Forest Laboratories with government fraud for illegally marketing its antidepressants Celexa and Lexapro for off-label use in children and teenagers and for hiding data that showed the drugs were ineffective and even posed a suicide risk for young users, and for paying kickbacks to doctors to prescribe the drugs, in the form of cash payments disguised as grants or consulting fees, paid vacations, baseball tickets, and gift certificates to pricey restaurants.

There has been an enraging arrogance behind these and other pharmaceutical-industry actions. There has been a really shocking degree of callousness and cynicism, whether in the Paxil ads that aired after 9/11 promising relief from anxiety while showing images of the collapsing Twin Towers, or in the boast of Vince Parry, a marketing executive who specialized in working with pharmaceutical companies and who bragged, in a much-quoted 2003 industry article, of how easy it had been for America's drug companies to master "The Art of Branding a Condition": "If you can define a particular condition and its associated symptoms in the minds of physicians and patients," he wrote, "you can also predicate the best treatment for that condition."

It was this arrogance, callousness, and cynicism that, by the end of the first decade of the 2000s, really defined the pharmaceutical industry in the minds of Americans, eroding public trust to a point where even industry leaders had to concede that their commercial practices had become self-destructive. "The drug companies completely shot themselves in the foot," a Virginia psychopharmacologist who ran drug trials for Eli Lilly—and believed deeply in the value of its drug Strattera for ADHD—told me, with a sigh of exasperation, in 2007. By 2009, there were signs that doctors were growing far more cautious about prescribing psychiatric drugs for children. Whether this is a healthy development, a sign that drugs are being prescribed more judiciously, or a negative one, meaning that kids in need of psychopharmacological help are being denied it by their spooked parents and doctors, remains to be seen.

The backlash against the practice of prescribing psychotropic medications to kids was inevitable, given Americans' crumbling faith in the pharmaceutical industry. What made matters worse was the sense, felt by so many patients, and parents of patients in particular, that, outside of industry, in our government, no one had been minding the store. That whatever safeguards should have been in place seemed to have slipped.

That whatever watchdogs were meant to have guarded American consumers seemed to have been asleep at the wheel. Or even worse, once again—were in the pocket of the drug companies.

This wasn't just an idle perception.

We all know, of course, about the millions of dollars in industry donations that keep our politicians flush in campaign funds. We all remember the uninspiring example of Billy Tauzin, the congressman from Louisiana who left Congress in late 2004 to take a new job as the president of the Pharmaceutical Research and Manufacturers of America, Big Pharma's biggest lobbying group, right after having led efforts in the House to pass the extremely industry-friendly 2003 Medicare Prescription Drug Improvement and Modernization Act.

The influx of drug money into our government, however, hasn't just been limited to politicians. Government scientists, in recent years, have been well contaminated, too. The Food and Drug Administration, in particular, has become severely compromised. Starved of funds and political support since the deregulation-loving Reagan years, it started, in the early 1990s, building relationships with drug and device makers that, critics charge, have undermined its ability to perform its functions of guaranteeing patient safety ever since. In 1992, sorely lacking for funds, and pushed by AIDS advocacy groups to get new drugs to market more quickly, it worked out a deal with the pharmaceutical companies whereby they'd pay fees to the agency and in return have access to an expedited review process. Over time, the FDA came to rely more and more on these fees. And, critics charge, the fee-payers' influence expanded so greatly that it perverted the agency's consumer protection mission.

In 2008, Marcia Angell, who is now on the staff of the Division of Medical Ethics at Harvard Medical School, reported in *The Journal of the American Medical Association* that many of the members of the sixteen committees that advise the FDA on drug approvals have ties to drug companies. "Although these individuals are supposed to recuse themselves from participating in decisions about drugs made by specific companies with which they have a financial relationship, that requirement is frequently waived by FDA authorities," she wrote.

That same year, Senator Grassley, who as chairman of the Senate Finance Committee had oversight of the FDA, accused the agency of outright collusion with the pharmaceutical industry for relaxing rules limiting the dissemination of information on the off-label use of drugs and devices to doctors. "What the FDA once considered evidence of unlawful marketing/misbranding/adulteration of a drug or device, the Agency would now consider an appropriate dissemination of information," he remarked, in a letter to FDA Commissioner Andrew C. von Eschenbach that April. "In effect, the FDA is ceding some of its oversight of off-label promotion."

A number of chilling stories have emerged in recent years of whistle-blowers—scientists who strove to speak out against the dangers of drugs receiving FDA approval—being silenced and even harassed by the agency. One, Dr. Andrew Mosholder, a top agency epidemiologist, made headlines in 2004 when the story emerged that FDA officials had tried to prohibit him from testifying in a public hearing about his research indicating that antidepressants like Paxil made children twice as likely as those taking placebo to become suicidal. (He recommended that no antidepressant other than Prozac, which had proven efficacy in children and had not been linked to suicidality, should be used in children.)

In the wake of widely publicized stories like Mosholder's, the damage to the public's esteem for the FDA was profound. The FDA's failure to protect patients from dangerous drugs like Vioxx, coupled with the damaging revelations about the harassment and silencing of whistle-blowers, badly marred its image with the American public. Faith in the agency's ability to do a good or excellent job in protecting drug safety fell a full 20 percentage points between 2004 and 2006. In 2006, 82 percent of Americans surveyed told *The Wall Street Journal* they believed the FDA's decisions were influenced by politics rather than medical science, and another 80 percent said they were "very concerned" about the agency's ability to "make independent decisions that will ensure that patients have access to safe and effective medicines."

The frighteningly too-cozy relationship between government and industry hasn't been limited to the FDA and its scientists. In 2005, the National Institutes of Health were forced to turn themselves inside out to fight the appearance of drug money corruption, after the extent of industry infiltration of the NIH became known to the public. In the late 1990s, the pharmaceutical companies had established extensive relationships with top NIH scientists. Senior scientists were found to be padding their government incomes with large consulting fees and stock options from drug companies they were dealing with and helping in the companies' marketing efforts. Some earned hundreds of thousands of dollars in this way. The outside work was supposed to be approved by superiors, and scientists were supposed to recuse themselves from decisions affecting the companies they were consulting for. But most did not have to file disclosures on outside income.

As was the case at universities, which were supposed—and commonly failed—to track which of their researchers were getting drug-company money and keep that money from comingling with government grant funds, the system of self-policing at the government agency simply wasn't working. In 2005, the NIH adopted strict new ethics rules barring scientists at the agency from consulting with private industry, prohibiting high-level scientists from owning shares in pharmaceutical and biotech companies, and even from accepting many academic prizes.

As the NIH made these changes, there was a certain amount of handwringing on the part of scientists, who worried that the "best and brightest" in their midst would be forced out of the public sector because of the blow to their now expected levels of compensation. The pull of big money had just become inescapable in the decades following the Reagan Revolution, when legislative changes made it possible, for the first time, for academic researchers to make big money from their discoveries. It was a cultural shift, and it reached its apex around the turn of the millennium. As our country hurtled toward financial disaster, science was corrupted by the lure of outsized rewards, much as was the unregulated financial industry. "Greed became respectable," Angell told me in the fall of 2008, as the markets melted down. "There was a strong feeling that the world divided into winners and losers. In medical research this just has had enormous implications."

In the area of children's mental health, the implications of all this are profound: Parents feel like they have no one in the medical profession to turn to for unbiased information, and no one in the government reliably looking out for the safety of their children. There are, of course, excellent and trustworthy doctors and government scientists of great integrity. But how to know who to trust, when you sit in doctors' waiting rooms elbow to elbow with drug reps? How safe can one feel when the brochure your doctor hands you to explain the action of the medication your child has just been prescribed was written by the drug's maker? How much faith can you have in research that bears the imprimatur of industry?

The greed and opportunism that bind some doctors way too close to Big Pharma aren't by any means unique to psychiatry. But they have had a uniquely damaging effect on a specialty that has for so long been contested and controversial. (Psychiatry, Thomas R. Insel, director of the National Institute of Mental Health, told me, "is the only field where the doctors are more stigmatized than the illness.")

For many people, the revelations of psychiatry's extensive ties to the pharmaceutical industry are just proof of the inner corruption of the whole psychiatric enterprise in the age of biological psychiatry, or, as critics call it, "blaming the brain." I saw this very clearly when I wrote for *The New York Times* in October 2008 about Dr. Nemeroff, the Emory University psychiatrist who, it turned out, had made millions of dollars consulting for up to twenty-one drug and device companies simultaneously. Immediately, readers jumped in to say that such ties to industry were just a superficial symptom of the deeper pathologies of Nemeroff's profession.

"While greed seems to have had something to do with this, I think that the root cause is the hubris of drug companies and researchers that somehow with our minimal understanding of brain chemistry we could create a magic pill for each of the mental disorders," was a typical response.

America's profound distrust and dislike of psychiatry didn't start with the revelations of the profession's corruptive ties to Big Pharma. They go much deeper. The very practice of psychiatry in its current biological form is for many people anathema—antithetical to their deepest views of what should constitute true emotional caretaking, contrary to profound and basic beliefs about what it is that makes us human and what it should take to make us well.

These beliefs are particularly acute when it comes to children, because of their vulnerability, because their brains are still developing, because there is still so much resistance to the idea that kids really can have psychiatric issues that are more than the normal vicissitudes of growing up, or do have problems that are more than normal reactions to our "crazy" times.

The current paradigm for treating kids with medication, which basically consists of medicating symptoms in the hope that, with their symptoms erased or attenuated, children with mental health issues can go on to develop more normally and learn, play, and grow emotionally like other kids, is for many an offensive notion. The old Freudian belief that symptoms are superficial, that the true work of any kind of therapeutic intervention has to be to reach deeper, to get at the "real" psychic conflicts operating behind them, still has a powerful hold on most people's minds. That is why there still is so much opposition—outside and to some extent within the mental health establishment—to the view of mental ailments as "brain disorders." For many psychologists, social workers, and many members of the lay public, the brain-based explanation continues to feel like a cop-out, chemical treatment a band-aid at best. For people who believe this deeply, the notion of treating children in this way is nothing less than criminal.

Yet the sense that psychiatry is a corrupting force, aimed at changing and controlling the very essence of human nature, far predates the use of psychotropic medication to treat children. In fact, when it comes to our nation's fears about psychiatry, the "drugging children" debate is just the tip of the iceberg.

· 7 ·

Stuck in the Cuckoo's Nest

"Right now, if the statistics are correct, about 15 percent of Americans are not happy. Soon, perhaps, with the help of psychopharmaceuticals, we shall have no more unhappy people in our country. Melancholics will become unknown.

"This would be an unparalleled tragedy, equivalent in scope to the annihilation of the sperm whale or the golden eagle. With no more melancholics, we would live in a world in which everyone simply accepted the status quo, in which everyone would simply be content with the given. This would constitute a dystopia of ubiquitous placid grins . . . a police state of Pollyanas, a flatland that offers nothing new under the sun. Why are we pushing toward such a hellish condition?"

ERIC G. WILSON, *AGAINST HAPPINESS*

As I was writing this book, there arrived in the mail almost weekly, it seemed, someone else's book detailing all that is wrong with modern psychiatry.

There was Wake Forest University English professor Eric Wilson's *Against Happiness*, an anti-antidepressant *cri de coeur* that warned that "the American obsession with happiness . . . could well lead to a sudden extinction of the creative impulse, that would result in an extermination as horrible as those foreshadowed by global warming and environmental crisis and nuclear proliferation."

There was Northwestern University Victorian literature scholar Christopher Lane's book *Shyness: How Normal Behavior Became a Sickness*, which decried how antidepressants have caused a "widespread emotional blunting—altering the strength of our attachments, how well we can concentrate, and even how deeply we fall in love." ("The sad consequence," he writes, "is a vast, perhaps unrecoverable, loss of emotional range, an impoverishment of human experience.")

There was writer Charles Barber's *Comfortably Numb: How Psychiatry Is Medicating a Nation*, inveighing against the age of The Medicated American ("A certain measure of depression is absolutely appropriate to this world. Indeed, it can be a sign of health, an indicator of being a thinking, feeling person—proof that one is alive," he writes).

There were Brandeis University sociologist Peter Conrad's *The Medicalization of Society: On the Transformation of Human Conditions into Treatable Disorders*, and sociology and social work professors Allan V. Horwitz and Jerome K. Wakefield's *The Loss of Sadness: How Psychiatry Transformed Normal Sorrow into Depressive Disorder*.

The books that crossed my desk weren't, with the exception of John Rosemond and Bose Ravenel's *The Diseasing of America's Children*, specifically focused on kids. (Though Lane did give a nod to that most common and most contested disorder of childhood, ADHD: "'We used to have a word for sufferers of ADHD. We called them *boys*,'" he quotes a psychoanalyst's lament.)

Their basic arguments, however, neatly paralleled the key elements of the Medicated Child story line: Vast numbers of normal, healthy people, the books asserted, are now being drugged into emotionally blunted submission. Psychiatrists—"bright and ambitious people" who "devote their lives to erasing selfhood in order to cure it of its discontents," as psychotherapist Gary Greenberg wrote in *Harper's* in 2007—are now overdrugging essentially normal people, evening out the national temperament, using medications as "political sedatives," to borrow a phrase from *The New York Review of Books'* Frederick C. Crews, and in so doing muting whatever social protest or potential dissent malcontented people might raise about the unacceptable conditions of their lives.

The worry that psychiatry, "the arbiter of normality," as Allan Horwitz once put it, is "changing what it means to be human," to quote from journalist Ray Moynihan and policy researcher Alan Cassels's 2005 book, *Selling Sickness: How the World's Biggest Pharmaceutical Companies Are Turning Us All into Patients*, runs through all the rhetoric about child-drugging, too.

"How can we generalize normal for all people?" wondered a sociology professor, writing to *The New York Times* in 2007, about how "we overdiagnose and overprescribe psychopharmicological drugs to our young children."

> *"Is normal sitting perfectly still for 7 hours and never speaking, being totally willing to subjugate oneself to authority, never to speak your mind, conform to the fullest extent of the term in any given situation and to be happy as Barney 24/7? Give me a freakin' break! But hey, that is what seems to me that people expect of children in school these days. Is the bureaucratic lifestyle that we socialize children in beneficial for them? No. Is it perhaps even harmful? Yes. . . . Remember, mental illnesses are human creations, we define what is normal and therefore abnormal and we place definitions on conditions and give them legitimacy in some way, and because we ourselves are not perfect, as some would like to think, maybe our social creations are flawed as well."*

"Because our society insists that all children receive more or less the same kind of education ('No Child Left Behind')," the President's Council on Bioethics more solemnly warned, "we tend to ignore important individual differences and instead tend to treat difficult or non-conforming children as problems." Psychotropic medication, the council's 2003 report, *Beyond Therapy*, cautioned, may bring "an enhanced ability to make children conform to conventional standards."

Like the beliefs that underlie the child-focused part of today's Med Scare, the arguments about adults are expressed with a vehemence that is way disproportionate to their grounding in fact. It is true that large numbers of adults take psychotropic medication—particularly antidepressants: In any given month, about 10 percent of Americans aged fifteen to fifty-four take an antidepressant for mental health reasons (as opposed to say, pain management). Given the perfunctory nature of so many doctor-patient encounters in the age of managed care, and the fact that many of the doctors prescribing psychotropic drugs are general practitioners who have not been trained in the finer points of making psychiatric diagnoses, it's inevitable that some people will end up taking medications that aren't meant for them and won't help them. There are undoubtedly some people who are taking antidepressants when they really shouldn't, when, for example, they're suffering from the kind of passing sadness or grief that doesn't qualify for a diagnosis of clinical depression.

But there's no evidence to indicate that any truly meaningful number of people are taking psychotropic drugs for trivial reasons. In fact, what evidence there is indicates that, as is the case with children, mental health disorders are quite common in adults and tend to go untreated. Adults generally do not want to take medication; many resist doing so until they've gotten to a point where their suffering is very severe. Many don't take their meds once they've been prescribed, or they start and then stop as soon as they're feeling better.

Barber, in *Comfortably Numb*, actually admits as much: Only one-fourth of people who start a course of antidepressants continue to take them for more than three months, he notes. "That's why you have trace amounts of Prozac in the Washington water supply," Thomas Insel, director of the National Institute of Mental Health once told me. "People get them and don't take them. They toss them." Treatment guidelines from the American College of Physicians recommend continuing antidepressants for four to nine months—or longer, for a patient who has suffered multiple bouts of depression—once symptoms have abated.

Of course, we've all probably had the experience of hearing people say they're taking psychiatric drugs—again, usually antidepressants—for what sound like minimally troublesome reasons. But what people say in public isn't necessarily the most reliable indicator of what's really going on inside.

"People may say, 'I'm taking this [drug] to be a better writer,' but what you hear in cocktail parties and what you hear in the office is very different," Dr. Peter D. Kramer, clinical professor in the department of psychiatry and human behavior at Brown University Medical School, told me.

I had sought Kramer out in early 2008 to take up the issue of the trivial use of antidepressants because he's the person to whom accusatory fingers most commonly point when critics talk about the misuse of psychiatric drugs for personal "enhancement."

That's because it was Kramer who coined the fateful phrase "cosmetic psychopharmacology" in his 1993 best-seller, *Listening to Prozac*, a book in which he shared his reflections about the life-changing abilities of fluoxetine, the intriguing new green-and-white pill that was then revolutionizing the practice of psychiatry, surprising doctors with its ability not just to treat classic depression, but also, as he put it, to alter patients' personalities so that they became "better than well": more energetic, more "socially attractive."

Kramer has come, in many ways, to rue those words. Defending himself, fifteen years later, from charges that he'd ushered in an era of made-to-measure personality, he protested that he had only been musing about what hypothetically *could* happen in the age of Prozac. He had never expected, he said, that his "mnemonic" catch-phrase "cosmetic psychopharmacology" would be repeated over and over again until it became, in the mind of psychiatry's critics, conventional wisdom about his profession. "People were taking my worries about cosmetic psychopharmacology and applying them—in my view, mistakenly—to conventional uses of medication," he was still writing in February of 2008, attempting to set the record straight in response to Frederick Crews in *The New York Review of Books.*

When I asked him if he'd had many patients who'd come to him seeking medication for frivolous, "cosmetic," concerns, he was categorical.

"Not only have I not encountered many, I haven't encountered *any* in my office, or even in detailed phone calls," he said. "It's hard to be a doctor. You see a lot of sick people."

The many psychiatrists I've interviewed—and the many surveys I've seen—on the prevalence and treatment of adult mental health disorders echo Kramer's experience. But what the mental health establishment has to say means less than nothing to psychiatry's critics. As is the case with popular beliefs about children's mental health issues and their treatment, doctors'—and adult patients'—real-life experiences are largely irrelevant. Received wisdom is largely independent from truth.

The Med Scare—the now common conviction that psychiatric drugs are being used to control and denature normal and healthy children (and adults) who don't conform to society's expectations—is based more on fear than on fact. It is rooted not in a realistic assessment of what today's psychiatry is or does, but in ideology: for the most part, a modern vestige of old sixties antiestablishment thinking. (I find this impetus even in the thinking of conservatives like syndicated columnist John Rosemond or the intellectuals who made up the President's Council on Bioethics under the Bush White House. For them, the "establishment" being rebelled against is that of godless modern parenting and government meddling, in the form of public mental health screening and the encroachment of psychiatric concepts into the sanctity of parents' private lives and responsibilities.)

That these views are not generally viewed as ideological, that they have been repeated so very many times as to have taken on the appearance of fact, is unfortunate. Because it's one thing to have lefty literary critics (or right-wing bioethicists) engaging in the sterile enterprise of deconstructing society's interface with psychiatry; it's another thing altogether to have the results of these academic enterprises, trickle out, in decontextualized form, into our popular culture in ways that could affect how people actually care for themselves and their children. It's one thing to carry on the noble fights of the sixties—to fight "biomedical social control leadership," in the words of the crusading anti-meds psychiatrist Peter Breggin—and another to sacrifice suffering adults and children on the altar of ideology.

The opposition to medicating adults and to "drugging" kids springs, for some, from a decent-enough source: a desire to protest a world that's become inhuman in its pace, values, and demands, to avoid what some very deeply feel is the "stigma" of having a psychiatric label. (For psychiatry critic Larry Diller, I know, this particular fight has very personal roots. His parents, he notes in *The Last Normal Child*, were Holocaust survivors. "Their losses made me personally aware of the dangers of categories and stereotypes," he writes. "For me, the oldest child of Polish/Jewish immigrant parents, the potential risks of labeling someone as having a biological disorder are not abstractions. Growing up, I heard first-hand the accounts of people who navigated the nightmare of Nazi racial policies.")

But the antipsychiatry stance doesn't actually serve its purpose of protecting children at all. For one thing, it is too far divorced from reality. For another, it is too unthinking—a reflex now, for right-thinking people. Once linked to social realities, the antipsychiatry critique now exists largely independently of them, kept afloat by structures of thought that have taken on a life of their own over time.

Back in the 1960s, when today's antipsychiatry was new, there was good reason for protest. But the world has changed. Psychiatry has changed. There is still much to critique about the profession—particularly its excessive ties to the pharmaceutical industry. But without a sense of history, without a sense of the human dramas that lie behind all those prescriptions and "labels," and without an awareness, at least, of the ideological forces at play, the attacks on psychiatry are largely meaningless.

Psychiatrists weren't always viewed as enemies of human freedom. In the Freudian era, post–World War II American pop culture viewed psychoanalysis as a form of mental liberation, freeing up the spirit, throwing off the weight of repression, speaking truth to internalized power. In films like Alfred Hitchcock's *Spellbound*, psychoanalysts were often presented as brave explorers, leading their analysands on epic quests to find the truths buried in the recesses of the mind. Joanne Greenberg conveyed this vision precisely in her best-selling 1964 novel and later film, *I Never Promised You a Rose Garden*, based on the author's experience of being a psychiatric patient in the 1940s and early 1950s.

In the novel, Deborah Blau, a sixteen-year-old girl, lives in a parallel universe of her mind's tortured creation. Her psychiatrist's dilemma lies in coaxing her out of that parallel universe into a real world which, the doctor acknowledges, is one that any sane person might well want to flee: "It is only the choice which I wish to give you; your own true and conscious choice," the doctor says. In the end—and with the use of no drugs other than sedatives to get through the night—the patient recovers, thanks to the heroic honesty and creativity of the doctor, who was modeled after Greenberg's own psychiatrist, the famed psychoanalyst and Nazi refugee Frieda Fromm-Reichmann.

By the late 1960s and in the 1970s, however, in the popular mind, the psychiatrist was no longer a kindly figure on a quest for truth. He (for he was nearly always a "he") was a white-coated incarnation of The Man—an enforcer of social norms, a gaoler of free spirits, an agent of institutional power. The mental patient had become a celebrated agent of rebellion. Mental illness itself, many now believed, did not exist; it was just, to paraphrase Jean-Paul Sartre, a very human form of revolt against an inhuman world.

Much of the intellectual impetus behind this vision came from Europe, where, in the early 1960s, Scottish psychiatrist R. D. Laing had postulated that schizophrenia was a greater state of sanity than was life in mainstream society, the condition's signature retreat from reality essentially a sane response to insane situations. French philosopher Michel Foucault argued that "madness" was an invention of the seventeenth and eighteenth centuries, a trick of language that brought renegades and misfits under social control.

In America, the Hungarian-born psychiatrist Thomas Szasz, a professor at the Upstate Medical Center of the State University of New York in Syracuse, became the most visible face of the antipsychiatry movement in America. In books like *The Myth of Mental Illness* and *Ideology and Insanity*, he railed against psychiatry, and involuntary mental health treatment in particular, as a "pseudomedical form of social control."

"There can be no such thing as mental illness," he declared.

The writer who had the greatest effect on American popular culture, however, was Ken Kesey, whose 1962 novel, *One Flew Over the Cuckoo's*

Nest, has been a staple of school curricula for two generations, and has probably been the most powerful influence to date in shaping how contemporary Americans view psychiatry. The novel, and the disturbing 1975 film with Jack Nicholson, formed the nightmare point of reference that played in the mind of so many parents I spoke with about the agony they went through in deciding whether or not to medicate their children.

Set in a psychiatric hospital where the patients, with minimal therapy, are drugged, electric shocked, and even lobotomized into submission, it is a story of man against machine, the free, rebellious spirit against society's most oppressive and cruel forces of conformity. Randle Patrick McMurphy, a boisterous, larger-than-life personality who comes on the ward posing as a mental patient because he's trying to avoid having to do jail time on a work farm, isn't crazy, just a wild spirit who doesn't like to play by the rules. He shows no sign of mental illness whatsoever, but is given shock treatments and, ultimately, lobotomized, when he breaks too many rules and, in a righteous rage, tries to kill the coldly controlling, diabolically evil Nurse Ratched, who, by "dedicating herself to adjustment," has bound the men on her ward to her in toothless submission.

Many of us encountered *One Flew Over the Cuckoo's Nest* as teens or saw the movie when it first came out in the 1970s. We remember the book or movie's themes without remembering the details. Yet the details, if you feel like taking the time to revisit them, are highly instructive: There's a nasty degree of racism in Kesey's description of the sinister "black boys" who torture new ward arrivals with their prying eyes and predatory thermometers, and there's a disturbing degree of misogyny in the vision Kesey creates of Big Nurse Ratched, "a bitch and a buzzard and a ball-cutter," as McMurphy proclaims her.

You are supposed to take away from this the timeless message that psychiatry takes society's rebels and outcasts and mentally neuters them in order to shut them up and make them more tractable. But rereading *Cuckoo* recently, it struck me that the book is as much about mid-twentieth-century gender fears, and fears of male impotence in particular, as it is about psychiatry. The story is an interesting cultural relic, a remnant of an era when "Momism" was still perceived as a threat, but it's hardly an apt metaphor for understanding social forces at work in our day.

One Flew Over the Cuckoo's Nest belonged to its particular place, time, and context in many ways; Kesey had worked in a psychiatric hospital in 1960, at the height of the Cold War. He'd participated in government-sponsored experiments with psychedelic drugs, drugs that were indeed being considered for their use as agents of mind control. Like Chief Bromden, the faux-deaf Native American narrator on the mental ward, who believes a machine called the Combine is ruling his life, thinking people in Kesey's time were troubled by the effects that the demands of conformity, the machinery of the military-industrial complex, corporate America, and middle-class suburban existence could have on vulnerable minds. Kesey was also writing after a very dark period in American psychiatry. State psychiatric hospitals in mid-century had, in fact, been terrible places, holding pens for those deemed incurable by psychoanalysis, with care that ranged from grossly inadequate to downright abusive, and where treatments like electroshock therapy, lobotomies, and insulin shock justifiably terrified patients and the public alike.

Once psychiatric medications came to replace those brutal forms of treatment—a change that many hospital psychiatrists viewed as "liberating" for patients—there did come a period in which some medications, most notably the "minor tranquilizers" Miltown, Librium, and Valium, were too frequently and too lightly used. These weren't the kinds of drugs, like Elavil, Thorazine, and Lithium, that had emptied out the horrible state mental hospitals. They weren't medications that pulled patients out of psychosis or manic follies or unreachable depression; they just made life more livable.

They quickly became troublingly popular; the demand for Miltown, introduced in 1955, was so great that in the years after the drug came on the market, window signs like "Out of Miltown" and "More Miltown Tomorrow" proliferated in drugstore windows across the country. The drug was so popular in Hollywood circles that Los Angeles was soon dubbed "Miltown-by-the-sea."

In California in 1967, 17 percent of people said they made frequent use of psychotropic drugs—most frequently tranquilizers—and 30 percent reported some use of them in the previous twelve months. By the 1970s, in any given year, almost one woman in four and one man in ten had used a psychotropic medication, most likely a minor tranquilizer or a sedative. The drugs were, it soon turned out, highly addictive.

Concerns grew about the excessive use of psychotherapeutic medications in people who were not schizophrenic or manic-depressive, but just unhappy or overwhelmed with life or "anxious." (In the Freudian period, people who would today be called depressed were generally said to be suffering from "anxiety.") Social psychiatrists, their work begun in the traumas and pathologies of World War II, laboring in the postwar period to understand the ways cultural stressors could cause mental disorders, considered the new meds "a refined form of lobotomy." For leftist intellectuals, they were just a way to force people to fit the coercive mold of mainstream culture. For feminists, Valium and Miltown, disproportionately prescribed to women, and promoted by popular women's magazines in the 1950s and early 1960s as a means for dealing with irksome children, bothersome housework, and sexually demanding men, were hated symbols of women's oppression and of (male) doctors' tendencies to shut them up rather than hear them out.

There was much truth to the antipsychiatry critique of the rebellious period we call the "sixties" (and which really extended to about 1980). American society in the 1950s and early 1960s *was* normative and in some ways oppressive. The psychoanalysts' diagnosing habits were often quite vague, resulting in a lot of false diagnoses of schizophrenia (including, contemporary psychiatrists have argued, Joanne Greenberg's; had she been truly schizophrenic, they say, her miraculous—and permanent—return to sanity without the use of medication, would have been impossible) and an overuse of powerful tranquilizing antipsychotics like Thorazine.

Drugs *were* marketed in ways that confirmed all of society's prejudices: to calm "neurotic" women, re-empower harried men nagged by wife and mother; one 1974 ad for the antipsychotic Haldol (haloperidol), went so far as to feature a picture of an enraged-looking black man. "Assaultive and belligerent?" read the caption over his head. On the facing page came the text "Cooperation often begins with Haldol."

But the antipsychiatry movement—in its intellectual, pop-cultural, and, eventually, political forms—went further than merely critiquing the excesses and biases of the psychiatric profession. At root, it rejected the idea of mental illness entirely. And that is where today's antipsychiatry meets its predecessor. Its cornerstone belief is that there really is no objective demarcation between mental illness and mental health, that the lines between sick and well, pathology and normality, are "largely arbitrary," as Herb Kutchins and Stuart A. Kirk say at the outset of their 1997 book, *Making Us Crazy: DSM: The Psychiatric Bible and the Creation of Mental Disorders.*

And while some antipsychiatry writers now take pains to draw a line in the sand between those who are "truly" sick and deserve medication and those who are not and don't—with the exception of Thomas Szasz, who was still publishing books in 2008 with titles like *Psychiatry: The Science of Lies*—they tend to conceive of the deserving few so narrowly as to shut out in the cold anyone who was not a candidate for immediate hospitalization. ("Obviously, those suffering severe depression, suicidal and bordering on psychosis, require serious medications," writes Eric Wilson.) Depression that doesn't lead to suicide, anxiety that stops somewhere short of agoraphobia, obsessive-compulsive disorder that doesn't make its sufferer scrub his or her hands down to bare bone—none of these appear to qualify as medically treatable conditions; they are quirks of personality to be cultivated and preserved, perhaps even celebrated as expressions of individuality and highly refined sensitivity.

This point of view rests either upon utter ignorance of how painful and destructive symptoms that aren't life-threatening can be, a lack of empathy parading as intolerance for "whiners," or upon something much worse: a kind of sadistic impulse, a willingness to see people suffer, or, I suspect, in the case of antipsychiatry conservatives, a desire perhaps to preserve the natural order in which some—healthy—people are winners and others have to just deal with being genetic losers.

It leads, at the very least, to some very intelligent people saying some very stupid things.

University of Minnesota professor of bioethics, pediatrics, and philosophy Carl Elliott, for example, in his 2003 rumination, *Better Than Well: American Medicine Meets the American Dream,* ponders whether he ought to use Ritalin to rein in his daydreaminess and better please his German wife, for whom his absentminded inefficiency is a "Bad Thing." He is one of four brothers, "all of whom were raised in South Carolina, and who have an air of abstraction and carelessness," he writes. "When something breaks, we fix it with duct tape. We are all prone to forgetfulness and sloppiness. We tend to live in our own heads more than in the actual, physical world. We are more likely to get lost, to forget things, to lose a thought in midsentence, to stare blankly off in the distance for minutes at a time."

But, he decides, like deaf people fearful of the loss of Deaf culture in the age of cochlear implants, like anyone, in fact, committed to preserving human heterogeneity, he prefers his "laid-back, Southern aesthetic of shabby abstractedness" to such "enhancement."

Why should he change? Why should his brothers? All are successful professionals: He is a professor, two of his brothers have graduate degrees in philosophy, and the other is a psychiatrist. There is no sign in any description provided by Elliott that—beyond potentially annoying their spouses—the brothers are subject to any kind of disorder or impairment.

Entirely missing here—and in all writing of this kind—is the notion that there is a world of difference between unique personality traits that may be quirky, annoying, or charming, and actual signs of pathology. Or that the difference between personal style and pathology resides in pain, distress, and impairment.

Whether based upon ignorance or intellectual dishonesty or malice, the conflation of personality and pathology is a very harmful thing. Its effect on people who suffer from mental illness—or the parents of children who do—is vicious and stigmatizing, and its effect on our culture is nothing less than toxic.

The romanticization of mental illness—and these days, it's usually depression, not schizophrenia, that is singled out as a higher, greater, more authentic state of being in adults, while ADHD is similarly mythologized in children—is downright nauseating for anyone who has ever suffered from a mental disorder, or loved someone who did, or worked with people who labor to free themselves from the constraints of their conditions. It is so easy to sit on the sidelines and applaud "melancholia" or daydreaminess, or designate kids who don't function well in school "Indigo Children" whose quasiparanormal gifts don't belong in the classroom, if you are ignorant of the day-to-day realities of true mental illness. (Or simply so invested in your own fantasy world that you refuse to acknowledge anything that pierces it. Eric Konigsberg, writing in *The New Yorker* in 2006, depicted this kind of scenario hauntingly as he described the life and death—by suicide—of Brandenn Bremmer, a homeschooled child genius who'd graduated from college at age ten and at fourteen had shot himself in the head after complaining to friends that he was feeling isolated and depressed. His parents, with the encouragement of a child psychologist and her spiritual-healer husband, decided he had been an Indigo Child, brought to earth temporarily for the ultimate purpose of saving others' lives through his organ donations. Talk of his having been depressed, his mother said, was just misplaced "doom and gloom.")

I have been shocked, time and again, by how thoughtless otherwise smart people can be on this particular topic, how willing to jettison common sense and, frankly, decency in pursuit of the antipsychiatry agenda.

The most egregious example I've seen over the past few years came when the judges of the 2007 PEN Prison Writing Awards decided to laud praise upon J. E. Wantz, a sex offender in Salem, Oregon, for his essay, "Feeling(s) Cheated." Wantz is a man who was plagued from his teen years onward by "depression, never directly addressed," which "built up like a pressure cooker without a release valve," and "abominable" sexual thoughts about boys his own age. He committed his first felony at age eighteen. Once paroled, and plagued by "black moods and a return of invasive and disturbing images accompanied by thoughts of self-harm," he enrolled, at the advice of a counselor troubled by his symptoms, in a state study on using Paxil to control recidivism.

The effect of Paxil was "that of a beacon, illuminating a once-murky room," he wrote. It freed him from "torment and despair," resulting in a "new me." But when he cut down his dosage or went off the meds—as he did, repeatedly, when the medication proved too costly, caused embarrassing sexual side effects, or was replaced by a cheaper generic—he had terrible withdrawal effects that frightened him greatly and made him think that the drug's manufacturer had fabricated the drug in such a way as to make it addictive. He also read an article in *The New York Review of Books* questioning the efficacy and ethicality of SSRI use and came to wonder what degree of his own creative genius was being sacrificed to the drugs.

Finally, after a volunteer prison chaplain began to "rail against the demonic possession of those on medication," he quit taking his meds altogether. "What have I suppressed by taking this drug?" he wondered. "Have I been cheating myself out of my own artistic responses and temperament?"

One wonders if his depression returned afterward. And what of the "abominable" thoughts—and criminal behaviors? The prizewinning essay doesn't say.

Autism is another disorder that in recent years has been romanticized, transformed by some advocates, parents, and even high-functioning autistics themselves, from a tragic occurrence to a kind of a gift. Famous artists, innovators, and intellectuals are now retrospectively diagnosed as autistic, proving that the condition, rather than being a life-limiting disorder, can actually be a gateway toward genius.

Perhaps this kind of public relations work does enhance the self-esteem of some people on the autistic spectrum. Perhaps it makes some parents of autistic children, on some level at least, feel better. And yet, as Michael Fitzpatrick, a general practitioner, father of an autistic boy, and the author of the myth-debunking *MMR and Autism: What Parents Need to Know,* has argued, this mental trick can have real dangers as well.

"The vogue for identifying autism in scientists and artists of the past (Newton, Einstein, Warhol) and even among contemporary celebrities (Bill Gates) romanticizes people with autism as creative and 'interestingly different,'" he wrote, while reviewing a slate of autism-related books in July 2006 for the online magazine *Spiked.* "But," he continued, "autism is not simply a different—and more exotic—way of being that causes minor problems of adjustment. It is a profound disorder of development that creates enormous difficulties for affected individuals throughout their lives, even if they are among the rare few blessed with special talents. Though well intentioned, the depiction of autism as a higher form of individuality risks demeaning the suffering experienced by people with autism and their families, while downplaying their need for specialized services."

Ann Bauer, writing for Salon.com in April 2009, gave a heartbreaking account of seeing her idealized image of her autistic son come crashing down against the reality of his illness, as he changed, in early adulthood, into "something like a golem—bitter, rampaging, full of rage." Her son, formerly a "sweet, dreamy boy," began physically attacking her and brutally assaulting other women in the group home where, as he got worse, he had to live. As Bauer searched online for help and information, seeking to find out if other autistic boys like her son became dangerously violent in late adolescence, she kept coming across her own earlier essays, which had argued for seeing autism as a gift.

"For years I had been telling my son's story, insisting that autism is beautiful, mysterious, perhaps even evolutionarily necessary. Denying that it can also be a wild, ravaging madness, a disease of the mind and soul. It was my trademark as an essayist, but also my profound belief," she wrote.

Bauer began her essay with the story of Trudy Steuernagel, a Kent State political scientist, who was beaten to death by her eighteen-year-old autistic son, Sky. She ended it with an account of how, after her son nearly strangled a young woman in his group home, she'd acquiesced to all sorts of awful treatments—electroshock therapy, massive doses of different drugs—to guarantee that he'd never be a danger to anyone again.

After having resisted the impulse to kill herself, her new calling in life, she decided, "must in part be to break the silence about autism's darker side," she wrote. "We cannot solve this problem by hiding it, the way handicapped children themselves used to be tucked away in cellars. In order to help the young men who endure this rage, someone has to be willing to tell the truth."

The truth goes a long way toward explaining why some parents are willing to make decisions that to other parents would be just unthinkable: going before a judge to green-light electroshock therapy, for example, as Bauer had to do, or agreeing to let a child who wasn't having out-of-control rages be treated with a powerful and potentially dangerous antipsychotic.

A New York City man, whose wife had contacted *The New York Times* in horror after pharmaceutical-industry reporter Gardiner Harris had written on the excessive off-label use of the antipsychotic Risperdal for children with ADHD, told me of the sequence of events and worries that had led him and his wife to accept giving Risperdal to their ten-year-old daughter, who has Asperger's and "serious attention issues" that interfere with her ability to learn and to navigate life, generally.

The girl had tried a variety of ADHD medications and had no success, he said. When her psychiatrist had suggested Risperdal—which is approved for use in treating irritability in autistic children—the parents had agreed to try it, even though, the dad commented, his daughter did not have temper outbreaks or other irritable behaviors.

"We'd asked the doctor, 'Isn't this an off-label use?'" the father said. "He'd said, 'No, this is fine.'"

The parents were eager to trust the doctor. The father admitted that he'd once harshly judged people who took psychotropic medication, and, even more, people who medicated their children. He had once been one of the many who viewed medication use as child-enhancement. Having a daughter who had to struggle hard to learn, relate, and function had changed his feelings. To those who would judge him now, he says, "If you won the genetic lotto, why should other people born with a certain chemical or genetic predisposition have to tough it out?"

This family was lucky. Their daughter was in a special-education school geared toward her learning style. She was surrounded by other special-needs kids and sensitive adults who created an environment in which she could grow and thrive. But leaving the attention issues unmedicated—the parents tossed the Risperdal script just as soon as they read the *Times'* warnings about it and scrapped the psychiatrist as well—was leaving the dad extremely anxious.

"Maybe I worry too much," he told me. "Not so long ago, my daughter used to do things like pick up the phone and speak into the wrong end of it. Now she can do that. People say the prognosis for her is very good. There are lots of people who are very strange who do very well." But, he added, when he attends meetings that draw together special-needs kids and their parents, he can't refrain from looking around the room and doing the math: How old, he wonders, will the parents be when their kids hit adulthood? For how many years will they be able to stand by them, shepherding them through life and protecting them? How long will he be around to help his daughter?

"Her attentional issues are the things I've worried most about for years," he revealed to me. "I used to work in the criminal justice system, so I know what can happen to people. I always worry that she's prey."

Today's antipsychiatry has much to feed upon: the corruption of the profession by drug money, the erosion of doctor-patient trust. But it is also now, like a functionally autonomous symptom, largely ahistorical. The conformist, oppressive, hierarchical, patriarchal, paternalistic, racist society that inspired the revolts of the sixties has to a large extent changed. The vast bulk of the psychiatrists practicing today were trained either in the crisis period of the late 1960s and 1970s, when psychiatry was most directly under attack, or afterward. The profession is now aware of its shameful history and tends not to find within its ranks a whole lot of the kinds of people who would have conducted thought experiments for the CIA during the Cold War.

Psychiatrists are, frankly, the oddballs of medicine—paid less, respected less, perhaps less mainstream than their peers in other specialties. Given this, being singled out as the contemporary version of The Man is an odd fit.

Peter Kramer, a progressive who—eight years after *Listening to Prozac*—

published a novel in which a "very thoughtful" man goes around blowing up "trophy homes" on Cape Cod, says he feels this oddness acutely.

"Evidence aside, I think it [the antibiological psychiatry stance] is one of these cultural tropes that's just a marker of humanism or sophistication often without being right," he told me. "It draws on this science-fiction anxiety about rapid technological change and anticapitalism, fear of the excesses of capitalism—which, really, I share. In this culture, to be against these intimate technologies and pro-therapy or against both is the favored posture. To say the drug companies may be making a valid contribution or say that mental illness may be fairly common is like . . . being a Republican. I find myself," he said, "on the wrong side of where your gut wants to be."

But, he added, "I'm suspicious of this trope precisely because it puts you on the 'right' side of everything. The facts do matter, finally."

Facts don't have much sway when you're in the grip of a religion. And with its ahistoricism, with its passion flaring so independently from fact and lived experience, there is something almost religious about the fervor of antipsychiatry today. The psychiatrist Gerald L. Klerman identified this religious tenor in the opposition to biological psychiatry back in the early 1970s. He called it "pharmacological Calvinism," and found it particularly to be strong in nonbiologically minded mental health professionals. "Especially among psychoanalysts and other psychotherapists there is the view that any drug use is a 'crutch' and that the best way to cure schizophrenia, neurosis, depression is through psychotherapeutic means using verbal insight," he wrote in *The Hastings Center Report*, in 1972.

> *"The conviction is often held that the use of psychotropic drugs in psychiatric treatment is morally wrong, independent of its efficacy, because*

> *it promotes gradual dependency. Drug therapy is thus a secondary road to salvation; the highest road to salvation is through insight and self-determination. . . . Implicit in this theory of therapeutic change is the philosophy of personal growth, basically a secular variant of the theological view of salvation through good works."*

The secular theology of therapy is, perhaps, less powerful today than it was in the early 1970s. But it is by no means gone.

The antipsychiatry argument has remained in circulation for so long because it has a natural resonance in our culture, reinforcing certain deep-seated, quasireligious beliefs about who we are and how we function.

One of these beliefs is that there is a definitive mind/body schism that is inherent to what makes us human. We are not just brain function; there is an essence—call it mind, or soul, or free will—that distinguishes us as sentient beings.

Another is that we are who we are because of our personal stories. We are depressed because our parents got divorced, or anorexic because our mothers were controlling. Biological psychiatry challenges these stories that give our lives meaning. It casts doubt upon the deterministic importance of early experience.

And while all the psychiatrists I've interviewed say that you can't ignore experience, that it is simplistic and wrong to do so, that it plays a role, along with genes and temperament in determining who we become, it is not—with the exception of extreme experiences like abuse or trauma or neglect—the one and only cause of sickness. The now predominant idea in psychiatry—that mental illness is a result of a complex interplay of nature and nurture with no singular cause (and thus, no "aha! moment" of cure possible from talk therapy)—puts the lie to the idea that psychic truth will set you free. It runs counter to the very American notion that every problem has a solution. Successful drug treatment also upends the idea that change is impossible without strenuous personal effort. (Lasting change probably is impossible without the tough personal effort of good therapy, but some improvement is possible without it. Should people be denied that improvement, that relief of their pain, simply because it seems to come without soul-strengthening effort?)

If people get largely better via chemicals—as many do—it challenges the meaning of the narrative of our lives. It doesn't make personal history irrelevant—it would be simplistic to say that—but it certainly scrambles the elements of causality, destroying the hierarchies of meaning by which we've tended to organize our lives. ("The way neurochemicals tell stories is not the way psychotherapy tells them," Kramer noted in *Listening to Prozac.*)

Psychoanalytic theory was, in many ways, much better suited to the ways we naturally make sense of our lives. It was a teleological system where every symptom had a greater meaning, where every step led back to certain key conflicts, Oedipal, death-related, survival-related. It permitted a person to construct a story of self that had an origin and an end point: the promise of a cure, which could come when the whole ball of yarn of symptoms and defenses and unacknowledged conflicts would be unraveled and understood. In biological psychiatry, there is no such satisfying cure on offer, no promise that the truth will set you free. There is, in the short term, symptom management, and in the long term (for those lucky enough to be able to afford good therapy), the hope that, once symptoms are managed, new and better ways of living can be learned. "A person with mental illness can recover even though the illness is not 'cured' . . . ," states the 1999 Surgeon General's Report on Mental Health. "[Recovery] is a way of living a satisfying, hopeful, and contributing life even with the limitations caused by illness."

For those suffering from mental health conditions, symptom management may be quite good enough, or at least, in some cases, the best they can hope for. But for those looking in from the outside, symptom management seems a shallow, even a Pyrrhic, victory. A formulation like child psychiatrist Harold Koplewicz's "You medicate symptoms to get them through" can seem like a criminally superficial way of dealing with a child, a sign of doctors' willingness to conform to normative ideas of how one should think and feel. That's an issue that's raised every time a pharmaceutical company runs an ad selling, say, Paxil to dull the effects of the terror of 9/11 or marketing ADHD drugs as the modern-day equivalent of a mother's little helper. (I think here of ads like the full-page promotion of Strattera that jumped out at me from a copy of *Family Circle* that I picked up in a doctor's office in September 2003. "Welcome to Ordinary," the copy read, showing two boys holding up a model plane. "4:30 p.m. Tuesday. He started something you never thought he'd finish. 5:20 p.m. Thursday. He's proved you wrong.")

And yet, if you separate out drug ads from responsible psychiatric practice, if you acknowledge that mental illness is real, if you acknowledge that those who seek help from psychiatrists do so—at great expense, inconvenience, and under the weight of considerable stigma—because their pain has risen to a point where it has become intolerable to them, then the critique of treating that real pain shows itself for what it truly is: an academic, political, ideological exercise. An exercise deeply concerned with the human condition but relatively unconcerned with the trials of individual human beings.

This is all especially true in the narrative of the Medicated Child, which is the hottest flash point in the larger debate about psychiatry in our time. After all, no one is more genuinely authentic than a child. No one is, then, more at risk of being corrupted by the larger forces in our society, polluted by its norms. And no one is more vulnerable to the winds and whims of demagoguery.

The beliefs underlying the Med Scare gripping our country, and the Ritalin Wars in particular (I have come to use the phrase "Ritalin

Wars" in my mind as shorthand for the whole debate over diagnosing children and treating them with psychotropic drugs), have truly now become like a creed. And yet, they're only superficially about diagnosis and medication. They're only partly based in disapproval of today's children, disdain for today's parents, and distrust of psychiatry. For most people, they're rooted in a discomfort with our world generally. They're about a sense of menace bearing down upon our world, and upon the world of children in particular.

There's a sense that greater powers, profit-driven and amoral, are pulling the strings in our lives. There's a sense that childhood has, in many ways, been denatured, that youth has been stolen, that the range of human acceptability has been narrowed for our kids to a point that it has become soul-crushingly inhuman. Childhood, it's very commonly now believed, has largely gone off the rails. And there's something terribly wrong with the way that we, as a nation of families, are living our lives.

· 8 ·

Ritalin Nation?

"A fourth-grade teacher once told me, 'We'll have the biggest class-action lawsuit in history. They'll sue us for stealing their childhood.'"

WENDY MOGEL, AUTHOR OF *THE BLESSING OF A SKINNED KNEE*

In the late 1970s, Peter Kramer conducted some research for the Carter administration on whether or not American women were being overmedicated with Valium.

Kramer, like most people at the time, believed that "mother's little helpers" were being used to shut women up and keep them compliant. But his research, conducted with the help of the National Institute of Mental Health and other federal agencies, didn't back up this view. Women *were* being given a lot of Valium prescriptions, he found (as were men), because at that time antianxiety meds were being given—rightly or wrongly—as treatment for a wide array of problems, including depression.

But there wasn't evidence to indicate that these scripts were being written frivolously, or as part of an effort to stifle women's voices. The heyday of casual prescribing was long over. "It was patients with high levels of distress who had received medication, and high distress correlated with diagnosable illness," Kramer later wrote of his findings in the online magazine *Slate*. Further research showed that general practitioners were providing more "therapeutic listening" to women than to men, leading him to conclude that "prescribing did not replace 'quality time'" between women and their doctors.

Kramer also didn't find that there were great numbers of Valium addicts in the United States. In fact, there were some indications that—as is the case today with psychotropic medications—rates of prescription were outpacing rates of actual consumption of pills. And that, in comparison to countries like France and Sweden, Americans weren't taking that many tranquilizers at all.

"A quarter century later, the evidence about mother's little helpers is no clearer," Kramer concluded, "but the case can be made that what was at stake had less to do with medication than with society at large. Yes, Valium had its beneficiaries and its victims. But the broad trends now look to have had their own momentum—more conflicting responsibilities for women, less time with patients for doctors, and a loss of cohesion and gravitas throughout the culture. In retrospect, Valium supplied convenient metaphors for change to which it contributed minimally."

"The worries expressed about Valium were our worries," Kramer elaborated to me in a phone interview. "Women were being given these more diverse responsibilities, weren't being given their due, their voices weren't being heard, the culture in general had a sort of oddness about it, something was being covered over. We had a general sense of anxiety or unease, and these issues were being explained through the idea that we're just giving medication to women and not talking to them. All those issues found their symbol in Valium."

As it was for Valium then, so it is, I think, for psychotropic meds generally today. Prozac is now a metaphor for how unhappy life has become for many adults and how mechanistic and inhuman society seems. Ritalin is the Valium of children, symbolizing the impossibility of living up to the demands and pressures now put upon them, and the perceived need for them to resort to unnatural measures—"anabolic steroids for the soul," in the words of Steven Hyman, the provost of Harvard University and former director of the National Institute of Mental Health—in order to function. And the Medicated Child is the trope that brings together all of our diffuse worries about childhood in our day.

We live, after all, at a time when academic demands on children have been stepped up to levels that many adults find unnecessary and unhealthy. We live at a time when economic pressures are bearing down on families—and being felt and borne by children—in ways not seen, by the middle class at least, since the Great Depression. Largely because of these economic pressures, we live at a time when many families suffer from a sense of separation and dislocation, working long hours, distracted by worry, run ragged by the hoops they feel they must jump through to assure the next generation a shot at success.

Adding all this together, it really does seem to many people that childhood, as a time of relatively stress-free learning and play, has been stolen from kids, and an unnatural world of striving, isolation, competition, and pressure has been left in its place.

You see this sentiment expressed overtly sometimes, as in 2003, when the *San Francisco Chronicle* ran a series of editorials on the theme of "reclaiming childhood." (One editorial was entirely focused on the direct-to-consumer marketing of ADHD drugs for children.) You hear it all the time in the laments parents make that their kids don't have the unstructured time and freedom to roam that they knew as children. You saw it over the past few years in the vogue for nostalgic "Back to Basics" toys from the 1950s, 1960s, and 1970s, which sparked interest, in parents at least, at a time when the toy industry generally was dispirited and lagging.

Today's middle-class parents, particularly those raised in the 1950s and 1960s, sociologist Annette Lareau notes in her 2003 book, *Unequal Childhoods*, had young lives that were very different from those of their children.

Since the time of the baby boomers' youth, there's been, she says, a kind of "McDonaldization of society," with the freedom and ease of home life ceding to "rationalization," and an "increasing standardization . . . with an emphasis on efficiency, predictability, control and calculability" and a "logic of . . . impersonal, competitive, contractual, commodified, efficient, profit-maximizing, self-interested relations."

Lareau's view is that most middle-class families today enjoy this style of living. But I'm not sure that's true. A sense of melancholy, I find, pervades much of our parenting culture, coexisting with the frenzy with which so many families get and spend their souped-up leisure time. There is a sense that things are too busy, too fast. The demands of childhood are too much, too overwhelming. Childhood today, to most adults, just feels wrong: too rushed, too pressured, too atomized, too stressed, and too joyless. It feels too cloistered, overprotected, anxious, and anxious-making.

Whether or not it feels the same way to children is subject to debate. But there's no doubt that *parents* are worried about the effects of our sped-up, stressed-out world on kids. That worry, I believe, is at root what animates the current cultural narrative about the Medicated Child, which is only the latest in a long series of narratives Americans have spun, at times of stress, about their children.

As the historian Peter Stearns explains it in his 2003 book, *Anxious Parents: A History of Modern Childrearing in America*, those stories are often generated in our country in response to specific moments of acute cultural anxiety. They even follow, he says, a kind of "formula": "a legitimate concern . . . prompts a larger search for symptoms, which in turn easily is absorbed into the debate over the extent to which children are flawed and/or frail in the face of threats."

Right now there are many legitimate reasons to be concerned with our society and with childhood in our society in particular. The feeling that our family lives are out of whack has, as Stearns describes, prompted a search for symptoms, and while the most glaring symptoms might well be all the psychological wear and tear on parents (a host of recent research now shows parents today to be more depressed and anxious, less happy generally than nonparents), our culture has tended instead to focus on finding signs of pathology in children.

There's been plenty to find: anxiety, depression, eating disorders, cutting, out-of-control behavior, insomnia, all of which *at least in part* (more on that later, too) can be blamed on the onerous demands of our culture. But what has happened, as in all the other child "panics" that Stearn discusses (the fear of sexual predators, the fear of kidnapping, etc.), is that threats to children have been greatly exaggerated in the public debate. The vulnerability of children has been overgeneralized. A naïve view of what causes mental illness has predominated in public discussion, giving cultural toxins more power than they probably really have. And at this particular moment of stress, children with mental health disorders, particularly those taking medication, have been turned into symbolic pawns, instrumentalized in a debate over mainstream society's values and vicissitudes that, in truth, isn't about them at all.

As I think I've made clear by now, I feel that the "Ritalin Nation" point of view (I have borrowed the phrase from Richard DeGrandpre's 1999 book *Ritalin Nation: Rapid-Fire Culture and the Transformation of Human Consciousness*), which presumes that our crazy society is driving kids to distraction, creating the need for medication to control or anesthetize them, is largely wrongheaded. I feel it collapses the very real and important distinctions that exist between normal states of stress, anxiety, sadness, frustration, and anger that come about in response to our stressful, anxious-making, depressing, frustrating world and pathological states which are much more severe, disproportionate to life events, and have a life of their own that cannibalizes children's lives. I feel the "Ritalin Nation" view is overly simplistic and overlooks many recent discoveries in medicine that cast the role of the environment—parents, school, "society"—in a much more complicated light.

Environmental factors, psychologists and psychiatrists now agree, play an important role in determining what kinds of stressors or supports a child encounters in his or her life. But biology sets the stage upon which life events unfold, and remains a key player in a child's reactions to those events ever after. Although today's biological psychiatry is often caricatured as doing nothing more than "blaming the brain," in fact the dominant mode of understanding the role of biology is more complex. The main paradigm for understanding the interplay of genes and environment now is biology loads the gun, environment pulls the trigger. In other words, stressors, of various kinds, cause the gun to shoot, producing symptoms.

The pathologies of our out-of-whack society just can't provide a sufficient explanation for why some children develop mental disorders and the overwhelming majority don't. And yet I understand the impulse to see children with mental health issues as the victims, the "canaries in the coal mine" of our sick world. It was, after all, what I did until research and reflection convinced me to the contrary.

Believing that our toxic world is either producing symptoms in children or classifying them as abnormal when they don't conform is seductive. After all, there is so much wrong with the lives of children today. There is so much about family life that's deserving of the label "sick."

We live at a time of ambient anxiety and insecurity. Social insecurity. Status insecurity. Fear about the future. A large part of this is economic—decades' worth of wage inequality, a growing wealth gap, a lack of investment in and care for working families, now having exploded into a full-fledged financial disaster from which few families are privileged enough to be fully immune.

Poor families have, of course, always had to contend with toxic levels of stress. What's been new, in recent decades, has been the middle-class squeeze. The sense that people are working harder and harder and still receiving an ever-shrinking piece of the economic pie. (Which they are:

The average worker's pay stayed almost flat from 1990 to 2004. In 2005, while the economy was still "strong," more than 80 percent of American workers had seen their inflation-adjusted wages fall for two straight years and, for the first time since the Great Depression, Americans borrowed more than they earned.)

The basic comforts of a middle-class existence—a house in a good neighborhood with good public schools, health insurance, being able to save for college and retirement—have, in recent years, become luxuries for increasing numbers of families. Most families in America, thanks to exploding health-care costs and diminishing benefits, have in recent years been only one medical disaster away from financial ruin. Private colleges have increasingly become playgrounds for the well-off (a trend that appeared to be on the threshold of change in early 2008, with record-high endowments promising more largesse for the needy, until the bubble burst and universities' investments tanked). No community has escaped the scourge of foreclosure. No couple has escaped the sight of their retirement funds imploding. Not that they were having an easy time putting money aside for retirement before, the number of employers offering defined pension plans having fallen 20 percentage points—to 29 percent—between 1998 and 2008.

Whatever worries middle-class families were able to at least partially stifle—or defer—as they put music lessons, summer camp, and Gymboree on their credit cards—exploded into the open as the Bush years drew to a close. Overwhelming indebtedness became a crippling problem not just for parents but for college students as well. By 2006, recent college graduates owed 85 percent more in student loans than had their counterparts a decade earlier, and experts were estimating that about 40 percent of students were graduating with "unmanageable" amounts of credit card and student loan debt.

Once the economy collapsed entirely, the level of family financial worry was such that even the youngest children were exposed to it. Newspapers like *The Wall Street Journal* began running how-to features on explaining family financial strain to kids. ("Confirm for your child what he thinks he's already observing" was the advice from Stanley Greenspan, a professor of psychiatry, behavioral sciences, and pediatrics at George Washington University and author of *The Secure Child.*)

Anxiety—economic and otherwise—now permeates every aspect of our family life. There's status panic, achievement frenzy, competition gone wild. Fighting for what looks like a firm foothold on the future, families eye each other like competing teams, vying for prize money and medals. Kids' sports—an eventual possible ticket to a college scholarship or admission to an institution that might otherwise be beyond a child's reach—have been ratcheted up to such preprofessional levels that doctors are seeing stress injuries in children as young as eight, and the American Academy of Pediatrics, in 2005, was moved to release a statement warning of the physical and psychological damage that can occur from too early specialization in a sport. Families turn their schedules (and finances) over to managing kids' sports "careers." And kids, from the youngest age, learn to keep their eyes on the prize, with even sixth-graders, when surveyed, saying they're doing all they can to get into a top college.

At the same time, helicopter parenting, that anxious dance of "involved" parents with too much time on their hands, has reached insane proportions. Parents "co-play" with their kids in the sandbox, eager to raise their "PQ" (play quotient). Wealthy parents harass camp directors for daily updates on their precious charges' eating patterns and application of sunscreen, leading some "high-end" sleepaway camps to employ full-time "parent liaisons" just to handle such phone calls and e-mail traffic, "almost like a hotel concierge listening to a client's needs," as one camp consultant put it to *The New York Times.*

Separation anxiety appears to be as much a problem for fiftysomethings as for infants. Some parents stock up on spyware—buying GPS-tracking cell phones, wireless surveillance cameras, radio-frequency locator chips to sew into clothing—to keep track of their kids. Colleges offer orientation programs for parents who just can't leave campus on drop-off day. Moms and dads edit papers, buy textbooks to follow along with their college-age child's course syllabi. Parents of recent college graduates accompany their twentysomethings on job interviews or phone employers to help their son or daughter negotiate a raise. The boundarylessness can reach criminal proportions: In 2006, forty-seven-year-old mother Lori Drew posed as a teen boy and cyberbullied her thirteen-year-old neighbor Megan Meier after Meier dropped Drew's daughter as a friend. After reading a particularly cruel message from Drew, Meier committed suicide.

Yet for all the anxious enmeshment, true family togetherness is under assault on every front. We live, author and psychiatrist Alvin Rosenfeld has said, in a "connection deficit world" in which families compete and strive together, but rarely pause in their activities for meaningful conversation or downtime. Family dinners have declined 33 percent, and family vacations have decreased 28 percent over the past twenty years. And that disconnection from family, many mental health experts say, makes children and teens particularly vulnerable to anxiety and depression.

Although it's easy to blame parents (and kids) for this lack of connection, the fact is, most—outside the upper middle class—don't choose a harried and hurried style of living. Life chooses for them: American working parents now spend on average 350 more hours per year working than they did in 1979.

We live at a time when traditional family life has changed, yet no social structures have been put in place to ease that change for parents and children. For most families, the single-earner-plus-homemaker model is not possible (or, arguably, desirable); yet supports that would allow parents to better balance work and family are all but nonexistent. Nearly 40 percent of American workers have no access to the unpaid family leave guaranteed by the 1993 Family and Medical Leave Act. As of this writing, only three states in the United States require employers to offer workers paid family leave. Only 16 percent of employers offer leave with full pay now, down from 27 percent in 1998. And the percentage of employers who allow employees flexibility in moving between full and part-time work without a loss in job status has declined—to 47 percent—from 57 percent a decade ago. Fully three-quarters of Americans say they have no control over their work schedules at all.

In households where both parents work or the single parent works, nearly a third of children in kindergarten through twelfth grade are left entirely to their own devices in the afterschool hours. High-quality child care tends to be beyond the budgets of all but the most privileged families. In 2008, a study of basic living expenses for middle-class families found that, in the twenty states where public pre-K is only for low-income children, preschool was the single largest expense for middle-class families of four, accounting for nearly 30 percent of monthly spending. As of this writing, only eight states plus the District of Columbia were offering universal pre-K for four-year-olds. And most of the day care that exists is grossly inadequate.

According to the National Institute of Child Health and Development Study of Early Child Care, the largest-ever study of child care in America, only a quarter—at most—of the care provided at day-care centers provides infants and toddlers with "sufficiently stimulating experiences to promote healthy cognitive, emotional and social development," reports clinical psychologist Sharna Olfman in her 2005 book, *Childhood Lost: How American Culture Is Failing Our Kids.* Most centers, she notes, offer "mediocre to abysmal care." Low wages among child-care workers create great turnover in their jobs; a 2001 study found the teaching staff in child-care centers to be "alarmingly unstable," with 76 percent of teachers employed in 1996 gone by 2000. And poor quality day care, with large class sizes and frequent teacher turnover, a 2005 report found, causes raised levels of the stress hormone cortisol in preschool children, negatively affecting their developing brains.

Life for many older children is hardly less stressful. Almost half of

U.S. high school students said, in a 2005 survey, that they felt unsafe in their schools. Academic expectations have been edging up, starting at the earliest ages. Kindergarteners are now expected to know how to read, have mastered some basic math facts, and to be able to write simple sentences by the time they graduate to first grade. In some districts, kindergarteners are required to do as much as two hours of daily reading drills. Worried that their preschoolers won't be able to cope with the competitive demands of kindergarten, some public school parents have begun hiring tutors to get their kids ready for school. Prospective private school parents hire tutors and therapists to help their prekindergarteners acquire not only good fine motor skills, but organizational skills and "people skills," too. By 2005, one in five students at Kaplan Inc.'s Score! Educational Centers were between the ages of four and six. Kumon North America began accepting children as young as two for preschool tutoring. Homework has exploded for young children along with the raised academic expectations. In 1981, two-thirds of second-graders didn't have homework; by 2003 more than half of them did.

The Bush administration's No Child Left Behind initiatives brought a great push for testing and standards, but at the expense of all kinds of resources and supports that made school a more bearable experience for most kids. Lunch was cut around the nation to make room for increased academics. Approximately 30,000 elementary schools eliminated recess. The city of Atlanta, in 2007, even stopped spending public money to build and maintain playgrounds.

Reading instruction came to stress speed and a narrow definition of proficiency, with the result that other aspects of reading—for pleasure, or for deeper meaning, were sacrificed. By March 2006, 71 percent of the nation's school districts had reduced time for history, music, and other subjects in favor of more time for testable reading and math. Mentoring programs, offering crucial aid to children without supportive families, were cut along with other resources not specifically tailored toward teaching for standardized tests. Everything became geared toward making children more high-performing and competitive, in the narrowest possible way.

For middle- and upper-middle-class kids, life largely became an eternal college-admissions process. In 2005, the Philadelphia school district started offering some of its AP courses on Saturdays, so students could cram more into their schedules. Free time was all but eliminated—unstructured play replaced by team sports, various lessons, homework and, for most kids, massive amounts of screen time, with children eight to ten spending an average of 6.5 hours a day on television, electronic games, computers, music, and other media. (According to the Kaiser Family Foundation, 43 percent of babies *younger than one year* also watch television every day.)

All of this, chronicled almost obsessively in books and magazines and newspapers over the past decade, has contributed to a widespread sense that we live in a world where children *can't* thrive through natural means. Not in a world where personal trainers are being used by elementary school students to get a "competitive edge." Not in a world of $100-per-hour "enrichment tutoring" for good students eager to make it into the Ivy League.

Ours is, in short, a world where it's believed that any normal kid would pretty much *need* stimulants to perform as required, would need antidepressants to ward off loneliness and dislocation, would practically require antipsychotics to be dulled into something other than righteous rage. With life so unnatural, people wonder, how can a normal kindergarten boy make it through school without drugs, when he's expected to do seat work six hours a day? How can a normal preschooler survive long hours in day care with ever-changing providers?

Excessive homework, activities, and early school start times have created an "epidemic of sleep deprivation among adolescents," we read. Children as young as toddlers, studies show, now suffer from sleep deprivation, too. Children's use of sleeping pills—none of which are approved for use in those under eighteen—rose 85 percent in the first half of this decade. Prescription drug *abuse* by kids spiked, tripling among teens between 1992 and 2003—at a time when drug use overall was steadily declining.

A unique aspect of this new kind of teen drug use was that it didn't appear to be for escape or for fun, as in previous generations. It was about performance. In 2005, the Substance Abuse Research Center at the University of Michigan reported that "competitive" universities had the highest rates of illicit use of prescription drugs. "The goal for many young adults is not to get high but to feel better—less depressed, less stressed out, more focused, better rested," *The New York Times* commented upon the phenomenon.

The laundry list of ills caused by childhood in our society has filled the pages of our newsweeklies, newspapers, and parenting bookshelves for as long now as I can remember.

Disconnection—because of parental work, because of parental stress, because of every family member being locked into his or her private competitive hell—leads to depression. "Hyperparenting" leads to crippling anxiety once the nonstop parental supports are taken away. Lenient, boundaryless parenting makes kids self-centered, narcissistic, at-risk for anxiety and, again, depression. Lack of outdoor time causes attention and learning problems. Media use causes lack of imagination, passivity, lack of initiative, and attention problems. Excessive video-game playing may create a desire for constant entertainment, intolerance of boredom, difficulties in dealing with a world of real people. Excessive exposure to on-screen violence can lead to a desensitization to violence.

Early sexualization of girls—think "Hooters Girl (in training)" T-shirts for toddlers, and thongs for tweens—causes eating disorders, low self-esteem, and depression. Too-early academics cause high anxiety and lowered self-esteem, yield frustration and anger (remember all those preschool expulsions?) and produce out-of-control kindergarteners who can do math but have no social skills. An excessive value on success above all else and at all costs causes a lack of development of other human qualities like care for other people. Lack of free play and too much screen time make kids lack imagination and creativity. Overscheduling and constant adult surveillance impedes children's abilities to take risks and be independent. Lack of traditional games like hopscotch and jump rope lead to children with a lack of motor skills that land them in occupational therapy. Too much stress on competitive sports leads to eating disorders. The endless focus on achievement stunts the development of other values that would create balanced, empathetic human beings. And the college admissions process turns kids into "manipulative spin-meisters" who "feel like frauds."

The endless parade of titles—*Generation Me, A Nation of Wimps, College of the Overwhelmed, Last Child in the Woods, Running on Ritalin, Home-Alone America, Silver Spoon Kids, Born to Buy, Failure to Connect, Consuming Kids, The Pampered Child Syndrome, Ritalin Nation, The Hurried Child*—suggests a ravenous market for news about all the ways in which today's society is messing up today's kids.

I have no doubt that all the social pathogens detailed above cause "issues" for children (and for parents). They at the very least appear to be creating a generation of badly behaved kids, and self-centered, narcissistic, entitled young adults. College students who lack proper boundaries, and treat professors as stand-in parents, who are supposed to be at their beck and call. ("One student skipped class and then sent the professor an e-mail asking for copies of her teaching notes. Another did not like her grade, and wrote a petulant message to the professor. Another explained that she was late for a Monday class because she was recovering from drinking too much at a wild weekend party," *The New York Times* reported back in 2006.) Young office workers who are "pampered, nurtured and programmed," according to a *USA Today* chronicle of Generation Y.

Our collective issues may well have led many in the rising generation to be not very nice, happy, or good people. (In 2005, the Harvard University admissions office, in a rather extraordinary paper, "Time Out or Burn Out for the Next Generation," suggested that it's not only the most vulnerable kids who fall victim to the vicissitudes of a lifetime spent in the "frenzied search for the brass ring." The authors wrote, "Even those who are doing extraordinarily well, the 'happy warriors' of today's ultra-competitive landscape, are in danger of emerging perhaps a bit less human.")

But is being, say, narcissistic, immature, unhappy, soulless, and anxious the same thing as having a real mental health disorder? That is to say—a condition that lives up to the *DSM-IV*'s standard of a "clinically significant behavioral or psychological syndrome" that is "associated with present distress" and causes "impairment in one or more important areas of functioning" or "increased risk of suffering, death, pain, disability or an important loss of freedom"?

Can society *cause* these kinds of disorders?

The prevailing opinion among mental health experts now is that it cannot. Not on its own.

Clearly, our world is overflowing with stressors. And stress—beyond manageable normal life levels that build mastery and resilience—is a toxin. It changes the brain. In extreme doses, as with the deprivations of poverty, it has been shown to damage children's prefrontal lobes—the area that controls abstract thought, executive function, and problem-solving to the point where, in some areas of functioning, the children operate almost at the level of stroke victims. In less extreme doses, it can change children's brains, too, priming "the stress system so that it responds at lower thresholds to events that might not be stressful to others, thereby increasing the risk of stress-related physical and mental illness," the *Journal of Cognitive Neuroscience* reported in January 2009. Chronic stress is believed to lead to depression.

Yet the threshold at which stress becomes toxic—and the degree to which it is toxic—varies from person to person. Life's stressors affect different children differently. That's why, for example, although the

American Academy of Pediatrics warned in 2006 that a "hurried and pressured lifestyle" could be detrimental to children's mental health, a number of researchers have found that some children are thriving under the superstructured, ultra-competitive conditions which many of us find miserable.

The New York Times, surveying fast-track sixth-graders nationally in 2000, found that "Some of the students suffer tension headaches and bouts of anxiety, raising questions about the costs of growing up quickly. But a number of the students embraced this intense focus on the future, saying it gave more meaning and direction to their lives than idle hours in front of the television. They drink in the challenges like a first sip of coffee, a tantalizing if slightly bitter taste of adulthood." Dan Kindlon, in 2006's *Alpha Girls*, argued passionately that today's high-achieving girls were strengthened and empowered by their efforts to succeed. Joseph Mahoney, a developmental psychologist and professor at Yale, in 2006 surveyed more than two thousand kids between the ages of five and eighteen and found that most of them—even teenagers participating in more than twenty hours of organized activities per week—did not suffer from overscheduling. "A lot of the attention around overscheduling is, I think, in part focused by the outlook of a psychologist who sees children come in with problems of anxiety and stress, which is not something you can generalize to families in general," he told me.

Anxious and stressed children can become more anxious and stressed if they have a lot of running around to do; that doesn't mean that *all* children react to constant busyness that way. That's because life alone—with the exception of experiences of trauma, neglect, and abuse—does not cause mental pathology. Even traumatic events like divorce affect different children in different ways. Twin studies on the effects of divorce on children, for example, indicate that some of the negative outcomes may be less due to divorce itself than to inherited propensities for problems like depression—problems that can lead to a parent's unhappy marriage and divorce in the first place. There is even research now to suggest that lucky gene variants may protect kids who have undergone physical, sexual, or emotional abuse from the risk of developing depression as adults.

The message that's emerged from scientific research over the past few decades is that there is an interplay between genes and environment, where environment can bring on or worsen inherited or biological disorders. This complex and nuanced way of thinking opens up avenues for understanding that are very different from those dictated by the more black-and-white terms through which children's mental health issues are typically painted in the public debate. It suggests that, on the one hand, the blame game is idiotic: With the exception of cases of abuse and neglect, there's no way to say parents *cause* their children's mental health conditions. Large classrooms, boring teachers, unrealistic academic standards don't *cause* ADHD (though they can promote signs of frustration and restlessness that mimic some ADHD symptoms). Skinny models don't *cause* anorexia nervosa (though they obviously play a role in giving that disorder its particular form).

On the other hand, having a multifaceted understanding of the source of mental disorders makes clear that we, as a society, *have* to think about children's environments. New research on intelligence indicates that a child's genetic potential is unleashed or not unleashed according to the kind of environment in which he or she is raised. There is also research to indicate that there are ways to act against children's genetic vulnerabilities. Positive caregiving, for example, can mediate the effect of genes that make children particularly vulnerable to stress. Free play and "high quality family time" apparently can, too.

We have to think about the conditions that enable and worsen children's mental health issues and either aid or impede their ability to overcome them. And we have to do something about our current social environment because it's creating—even among "normal" children—some pretty big problems. These are the social trends you read about all the time: the kids with a sense of entitlement, of emptiness, who have difficulties with growing up, leaving home, and facing life's challenges, who have inherited a game-the-system attitude that leaves everyone feeling ripped off. "There is reason to worry," said Michael Josephson, founder and president of the Josephson Institute of Ethics, which, in 2007, conducted the survey that found that high school athletes engage in academic cheating at a higher rate than their classmates, "that the sports fields of America are becoming the training grounds for the next generation of corporate and political villains and thieves."

Edward M. Hallowell, the coauthor of *Driven to Distraction,* has described how modern life can make people look like they have ADHD when they don't. In "Overloaded Circuits: Why Smart People Underperform," an article which appeared in the *Harvard Business Review* in January 2005, Hallowell wrote how he had come to differentiate between ADD, "a neurological disorder that . . . can be aggravated by environmental and physical factors" and what he'd come to call ADT or "attention deficit trait."

"Rather than being rooted in genetics . . . ADT is purely a response to the hyperkinetic environment in which we live," Hallowell wrote. "It is brought on by the demands on our time and attention that have exploded over the past two decades. As our minds fill with noise—feckless synaptic events signifying nothing—the brain gradually loses its capacity to attend fully and thoroughly to anything."

ADT, Hallowell says, is caused at base by overload, by having impossible amounts of work to do and being haunted by the awful sense of the impossibility of getting it done. Fear is the greatest destroyer of attention, he writes, "because emotion is the on/off switch for executive functioning."

Hallowell was writing about adults. (He took up the topic of hyperdistracted adult life in his 2006 book, *CrazyBusy: Overstretched, Overbooked, and About to Snap!*) But it's easy to see how well his thoughts about ADT could apply to non-ADD kids, driven to distraction by the excessive challenges of their academically hard-driving days. The ADD/ADT distinction provides much food for thought.

If we live in a time when the brains of non-ADHD kids are shutting down from mental overload, if we live in an era when even our young winners are "a bit less human," then it's fair to say that normal life now is "sick." But that's using the word "sick" as a value judgment, not a medical category, and it's urgently important not to confound the two. For to do so does a real injustice to children with mental health issues and their parents, and also makes improving empathy and getting better help for those children and parents all but impossible.

After all, kids with mental health issues are not necessarily "sick" the way those who soak up all the worst aspects of our culture are: grossly competitive, materialistic, entitled—characteristics that don't, as far as I know, show up anywhere in the *DSM*. Parents of children with mental health issues are not necessarily anything like those ones we all suspect are driving their kids crazy. The parents I interviewed were generally struggling with getting their kids to read, write, make friends, to function, basically, like "normal" kids—not like superkids. A few laughed ruefully that the one advantage of having a child with mental health problems was that it kept the family out of the rat race.

"I've changed my parenting goal. I just want everyone to have a pulse. I just want my kids to make it to twenty-one with their egos intact," the Virginia mother of boys with Asperger's and ADHD remarked to me.

The mother of a boy with epilepsy and emotional and learning issues echoed the sentiment: "We don't have the luxury of worrying about total bullshit things. You're worrying about your kid making a friend and living through a seizure."

Why do we focus so much of our meddlesome energies on the outliers—the children with issues serious enough to require medication and whose problems go beyond mere unhappy reactions to a stressful or suboptimal childhood? Why instead aren't we looking critically at the "normal" children who are perhaps being groomed to become unhappy people?

It's so much easier to point fingers at a minority than to look at the great mass of children and have to seriously call into question whether or not we're raising them well, whether or not our own values are showing up in them as signs of dysfunction. It is so easy to speak ruefully of "childhood lost," so much more challenging to try to give our children what we think they've missed.

"Modern ideas about the innocent child have long been projections of adult needs and frustrations," Gary Cross, a professor of modern history at Penn State University, writes in his 2004 book, *The Cute and the Cool: Wondrous Innocence and Modern American Children's Culture.* "In the final analysis, modern innocence has let adults evade the consequences of their own contradictory lives." He suggests that, instead of projecting all our mental confusion onto children, we aim to find a "more mature resolution to the contradictions of modern life."

If vast numbers of children are turning out—not sick, but kind of amoral, kind of limited as human beings—then we really have to call into question what's considered healthy in our society. Doing so won't make much of a practical difference to the children with serious mental health conditions. But it would be a worthy shift of focus.

"Sick," after all, doesn't have to be the new normal.

· 9 ·

The Stories We Tell

One afternoon in October 2007, I was driving in my car, listening to "Marketplace" on NPR, while a group of tweens chatted in the back.

"Here's something that might make your ears perk up: Starbucks is now a 'family destination,'" the announcer Bob Moon said, introducing commentary from humorist Tim Bedore.

"For a few decades now," Bedore began, "we have been medicating our kids—to deal with ADD or hyperactivity—in order to smooth out their behavior. And to help in that effort, Starbucks is going to start marketing coffee to teenagers."

One of the girls was taking medication for the inattentive subtype of ADHD. She did not know that it was aimed at "smoothing out" her behavior. She prided herself upon her good behavior.

"What?" she said, interrupting the chatter to lean forward in her seat. "*What was that?*"

As a culture, we tend not to think much about the effect of the stories we tell about children with mental health issues. The offhand comments, the snide little jokes, the eye-rolling, knowing looks—"Well, they all have *something* now, don't they?" "Aren't we *all* ADD?"—they've all just become an unthinking conversational reflex.

It's time to put some thought into changing that. Because the stories we tell are not just mostly wrong (as I hope I've now proven), they also do a great deal of harm.

The bad child/bad parent story line, in particular, blames and belittles children and parents and reinforces our society's worst tendencies not to help those who are in need. It trivializes real conditions. It romanticizes pain and suffering, making it that much harder for people to feel justified in seeking help. It collapses the differences between bad behavior and disorder, or between normal unhappiness and levels of distress that signal a larger problem.

This trivialization, this collapsing of boundaries between normality and pathology, rests in large part upon a deep-seated tendency in our culture to reject the biomedical model of mental health disorders. That's a theoretical position which, I imagine, will continue to spark debate among psychologists, philosophers, ethicists, journalists, and psychiatrists for years to come. For now, however, the debate is affecting public opinion in an immediate and toxic way: sowing disbelief that mental health conditions like ADHD are real, and breeding distrust, dislike, and even disdain for some of the most vulnerable parents and children in our midst.

The widespread, unthinking trivialization of mental health disorders in our public discourse isn't just hurtful and poisonous, however. It can even be dangerous for children with mental health issues, if it leads their parents to minimize their problems and not seek help for them. (And it does: Studies show that parents who don't believe that children's disorders are "real" don't get their kids help, even when the children are visibly showing symptoms.)

Casual insult feeds stigma. And stigma, along with "the 'culture of suspicion' it creates," wrote a team of researchers studying the issue in the journal *Psychiatric Services* in 2007, are, for children, the "fundamental reasons for the continued, pervasive level of unaddressed mental health needs" in our country.

We like to believe that we live at a time when having a mental health disorder and seeking treatment for it are no longer stigmatized. Woody Allen and countless "disorder of the week" magazine covers are supposed to have put an end to the shame of "seeing a shrink." The age of the brain was supposed to bring an end to the second-class status of psychiatry, that too-subjective, unscientific bastard child of medicine. A National Institute of Mental Health report in 2001, listing the new advances in mind science, was full of hope, predicting that, in the near future, identifying "genetic and biological bases of emotional and cognitive dysfunction should help to alleviate the social stigma associated with poor mental health." But that isn't what has come to pass. Although Americans' attitudes toward getting mental health treatment have improved modestly since the 1980s, true public acceptance is still a long way away.

In May 2007, *Psychiatric Services* published a series of articles which detailed the results of the first large-scale nationally representative survey of public attitudes about children's mental health. The nature of the responses to this *National Stigma Study–Children* showed that there is still a strong sense of shame in our country attached to the notion of a child's having mental health issues, along with considerable prejudice toward children with such issues and their parents.

Many respondents to the survey said they believed stigma would result from mental health treatment during childhood. They just about evenly split on the subject of whether getting treatment for mental health problems could have "immediate and lasting social ramifications for children and their families." Forty-five percent said getting mental health treatment would result in rejection at school and 43 percent said that the stigma would carry over into adulthood. More than one-third (35 percent) expected parents of children with mental illness to experience self-stigma.

Why was it expected that children would be stigmatized if they got mental health care? Because to be diagnosed is to be labeled "bad." Potentially very, very bad.

Call it the Columbine Syndrome: Ever since the news got out that school shooter Eric Harris had been taking Luvox, an antidepressant, kids' mental illness and eventual mass murder have been linked in the public mind. Eighty-one percent of respondents to the *National Stigma Study–Children* said they thought children with major depression would be dangerous to themselves or others; 33 percent said they believed children with ADHD were likely to be dangerous. These sentiments were echoed, also in 2007, by survey research at Indiana University that found about one in five parents saying they would not want children with ADHD or depression as their neighbors, in their child's classroom, or as their child's friends. Almost 30 percent of parents said they would not like their child to become friends with a child who was depressed, while more than 18 percent said they wouldn't want to live next door to a family with a depressed child. Almost a quarter of parents said they would not want their child to be friends with a child who showed behaviors typical of ADHD and slightly more than a fifth said they wouldn't want to live next door to a family with a child with ADHD.

It doesn't matter that there is little data to show that children with mental health conditions are particularly dangerous. (Unless they don't get treatment and begin self-medicating with illicit substances, at which point they can pose dangers to themselves and others.) What data does anyone need, when we have Harris, or Seung-Hui Cho, the profoundly disturbed Virginia Tech shooter who killed at least thirty people and wounded seventeen others before killing himself in April 2007? "Evidence suggests only a modest relationship between mental disorder and violence, a relationship that is largely attributable to co-occurring substance abuse," a team of stigma researchers noted in *Psychiatric Services* that May, with a sad nod to the "sensationalized media reports" and "(typically uninformed) inferences" that lead the public to fear young people with mental health conditions. "Unfortunately, public perceptions that mental illness and violence go hand in hand may be more important than evidence."

The stigma of danger surrounding children with mental health issues is easy enough to understand, given the enormous media attention that has been paid to mentally ill young murderers like Harris and Cho. But why, in the public mind, are *parents* expected to feel bad about themselves if they seek help for their kids?

Because to have a kid with mental health problems is to be a bad parent. "Many people in the United States embrace popular representations of childhood depression," for example, "as resulting from poor parenting—an attitude that stigmatizes families and creates barriers to care," the authors of a report interpreting the *National Stigma Study–Children* wrote in *Psychiatric Services.*

The negative attitudes toward parents of children with mental health issues showed up strongly again in another of the study's findings: that many respondents favored "legally mandated" treatment for depressed children. This finding was, on its face, surprising, given that so many people appeared to feel that psychiatric treatment was, essentially, a bad thing for kids. (More than two-thirds had "negative sentiments" about the effects of psychiatric medications on children.) Yet, it fit a larger picture of distrust and disrespect of parents. The public's stated views in favor of legally mandated care, the authors of an article on "Perceived Dangerousness of Children with Mental Health Problems and Support for Coerced Treatment" noted drily, "appear to reflect . . . the public's concern for parental responsibility."

Not surprisingly, because of stigma, and fears of stigma, many parents of children with mental health disorders won't seek services. They don't want their kids "labeled," even if a label is the ticket toward care. Even parents of children with mental health issues who end up in jail have been known to refuse psychiatric care for their children out of fear of the stigma of "labeling."

"They consider it a scourge," an Indiana circuit-court judge involved with a state pilot program aimed at moving mentally ill kids out of jail and into treatment said of those parents.

The parents in my research were well acquainted with stigma. They encountered it in other parents' attitudes all the time. Sometimes it took the form of fear based on ignorance. And sometimes there was fear of infection. "Other parents said outright they didn't want their kids playing with the special-needs kids," one parent of a former special-needs student in Washington, D.C.'s, most prestigious preschool told me, still angry, years later, about the limits of the school community's much-vaunted "inclusiveness."

Sometimes that particular fear of infection arose not because a child with mental health issues was so foreign to the fearful parent, but because he or she was too familiar—with behaviors way too similar to those of the fearful parent's own child. Sometimes one mother's decision to face her child's problem head-on was more than another mother could bear.

A Washington, D.C., woman told me of how she'd run into a mother she knew in the waiting room of a local speech and occupational therapy center. She happily told the other mother that her son, who has Asperger's, had just been admitted to a local private school that welcomes children with learning issues. The other mother was aghast. "Aren't you worried about the stigma?" she exclaimed.

"She was minimizing her child's issues," the woman told me. "She probably was terrified her child would turn out to have something. In my experience," she added, "this fear of stigma is more destructive than the stigma itself."

Often enough, in seeking help for their children, mothers—and it generally was mothers who sought help, at least at first—had to start by facing their own preconceptions, prejudices, and fears.

"Before my son was diagnosed, when I heard 'paranoid schizophrenic,' I thought, 'This is a violent criminal who's going to do me harm,'" a Pennsylvania woman told me of her psychotic son, who is a "gentle soul . . . when he's on his meds."

"In the past, when someone was manic-depressive, they couldn't be helped very much and you saw so much bizarre behavior that it was really scary," a Connecticut mother of a bipolar teen told me. "I worked after college for someone who was manic-depressive. I had a problem of someone stalking me from college; it turned out that he was bipolar. When I found out about my daughter's diagnosis, I was so upset. But the psychiatrist was so calm and reassuring and good about talking to me about the stigma. Over a few months, I felt so much better. For her, it wasn't this stigma, it was a chemical imbalance, and we could change it."

Many mothers described coming to terms with their child's diagnosis as a process akin to "mourning." They had to adjust their expectations of what their life with that child was going to be and learn to accept a new vision of who their child really was. "We all have an image of a child when we're pregnant, and when you get the diagnosis you almost have to go into mourning because you have to bury that child," the mother of a boy with Asperger's told me. "But you realize that you wouldn't have the child you do if you had that other fictional child. I don't want some fictional child, I want my son."

Once they did that, they often felt a great sense of relief. "One way to see autism and related diagnoses," said a Virginia woman with a son with Asperger's, "is to liken them to a European trip. You plan and plan your trip to Italy and you know exactly what to expect when you get there. However, your plane lands in France, which is still a great country and full of promise and great things to see and do. It's just not what you were expecting. So I'm learning to speak French."

Learning to speak this other language of acceptance and changed expectation was often harder for the fathers than the mothers.

"When we received Julia's diagnosis of autism, my wife kept repeating, like a mantra, 'There must be a reason for this. Everything happens for a reason,'" the writer Bob Berger wrote, in an article called "A Journey Toward Hope" in *Parenting* magazine. "I fell into a bottomless pit. . . . I began hating other families with normal children. Pregnant women with their dreamy, hopeful looks made me mad. I wanted the perfect little girl who stared up at me with curiosity and wonder just six months ago."

What was a mourning process for mothers was, for fathers, often a period of inner rage and retrenchment. Many refused, at least at first, to have their children "labeled." Many felt their wives were being duped by too-eager doctors. Many were highly skeptical about the value of therapy, highly suspicious of drugs, and, frankly, greatly annoyed with their wives for having gone down the road of "pathologizing" their kids in the first place. When acceptance came for these dads, it wasn't easy and often it wasn't total. Some put up passive resistance to the mothers' efforts—going along, but only so much. Others withdrew into themselves, entering a private hell that their wives couldn't access.

"My husband was in a difficult place," one New Jersey wife recalled of the period when she herself was "grieving" her daughter's autism diagnosis and throwing her energies into finding top-notch therapy for her. "Who takes this news lying down? But he took it really hard. He never saw the good side of what progress she made. If she was able to string three words together, he was always comparing her to typical kids. He couldn't appreciate or enjoy it because he was so devastated. I couldn't comfort him and he couldn't comfort me."

Over and over again, I heard in my research how fathers were particularly sensitive to the issue of stigma—and particularly resistant to seeking help for their children as a result.

"For my husband, [our son] is a mirror of who we were and are," a Washington, D.C., mother, whose son has ADHD and OCD and attends a specialized school for children with learning issues, told me. Getting her son diagnosed and treated for his issues was a long and hard journey, she said, made particularly difficult by the fact that the boy's father, a highly successful businessman, didn't want to see the problems. "My husband would be on board sometimes and sometimes not at all. I'd think he'd understand and then to my total surprise realize that he didn't. He blocked any kind of treatment for the OCD," she said.

> *"It finally got to a point where my husband was on a trip, my son was having a terrible flare-up of OCD about his father dying, needing to do terrible repetitions to keep his father from dying, from going down in the plane. My husband was on a trip he didn't need to be on, it was for fun. For two months. I called and told him, by blocking his care for OCD, this is neglect."*

When I spoke to the mother, the couple was divorcing. Their son, a high school senior set to attend a small liberal arts college in the fall, was on medication for his OCD. She was relieved that he was going to college, she said. But, she told me, "My son is down on himself in some ways. It's hard when you've got a father who doesn't accept you. It's really hard to feel good about yourself. Ultimately, I feel he could be in a much better place if we'd all been on the same page."

The mother I mentioned in Chapter 2, whose little boy told her he had to wear a certain pair of shoes to keep her from dying on any given day, faced similar resistance from her husband when she decided to seek mental health care for their son.

"I said to my husband, 'I have to find a psychologist or psychiatrist for him.' My husband said, 'I don't think I feel comfortable with our son seeing a psychologist or psychiatrist.' I said, 'You'd better get comfortable with it, because it's happening.'"

"I think he wanted to sweep it under the rug," she continued.

> *"That's how he was raised. The thought of seeing a psychologist–he thought [our son] could snap out of it. We could say that's ridiculous and he'd be fine.*
>
> *"I brought home a lot of reading material. I educated my husband. Now he's a lot more comfortable. But he's never met our son's psychologist. He's met the psychiatrist because the psychiatrist wouldn't prescribe medication without meeting both parents. I think the whole idea that his son had a mental illness is so hard for him."*

The mother of the bipolar teen in Connecticut also said that her efforts to involve her husband in their daughter's care could only go so far. "My husband has sort of left it up to me," she said. "He just basically has been, like, 'I know you'll take care of it right.'" Her voice went flat. "He hasn't been too involved."

While nearly all the mothers told me of the enormous relief it was for their children, after years of confused struggles, to be diagnosed and treated, one mother told me of a child for whom the stigma of being "labeled" felt like a death sentence. She was the African-American single mother in North Carolina who'd labored so hard to make sure that teachers and school officials recognized her son's difficulties and responded appropriately. When her son was in elementary school, she'd agonized about her decision to put him on Ritalin.

Then, when he was in middle school, she'd had the further heartbreak of watching him refuse to continue to take medication, and lose the ground he'd slowly gained.

"The first year of high school was an absolute disaster," she told me. "He went through a major, major depression. He decided he did not want to be labeled ADHD, he was not taking his meds, skipping school, getting into fights, was suspended. He had two hospitalizations—for depression. For suicidal ideation—he swears he was kidding around, but nobody was willing to take the chance. He became an angry young man because, one, he was hospitalized and, two, he was put on medications and felt he was being labeled. He was such a miserable kid, but he didn't want to be labeled or on medication. Now he still won't accept that he suffers from depression or ADD."

For fear of stigma, or out of self-stigma, kids don't get treatment. And without treatment, they don't get better. This isn't just a matter of getting a few bad grades or having a miserable year or two of high school. "Stigma has been shown to have devastating effects on the psychological, emotional, and social development of children with mental disorders, significantly diminishing their life chances as adults," the authors of a study on public attitudes and stigma concluded in *Psychiatric Services*.

There are real costs to not treating mental health issues. The risk of violence, however small statistically, is, of course, one of them, though private tragedies are far more common than grand acts of mass murder. One of the worst stories I've encountered came from *The Wall Street Journal*, which in August 2008 described the case of William Bruce, a twenty-four-year-old paranoid schizophrenic who was released from a psychiatric hospital in Augusta, Maine, after his taxpayer-funded patient advocates made the case that he did not need inpatient treatment or even medication. Though his doctors had judged him "very dangerous indeed for release to the community," Bruce was let go at the end of a court-ordered commitment term and returned to his parents' home, where he began hiding knives in his bedroom and spending days on end pacing and talking to himself in the driveway. Two months later, he killed his mother with a hatchet while she worked at her desk. He later told a psychologist that the Pope had ordered him to do so because she was involved with al Qaeda and Saddam Hussein.

Committed afterward, indefinitely, he began to take an antipsychotic. "None of this would have happened if I had been medicated," he later told the *Journal*. "The guilt is . . . tough."

Such violence is very rare. But what of the lives wasted, the potential squandered, the decades of unhappiness, the misery visited upon other family members by untreated parents and children with more common and less obvious forms of mental illness?

"My mother has OCD and is in total denial about it," said the mother of the boy who believed his shoes could save her life. "She's such an incredible worrier. I think she could have had such a happier life if she'd gotten help or medication. Instead, she tried to self-medicate.

> *"For years, she abused alcohol. She became a raging alcoholic. Once when my father was away, I picked up my four-year-old sister, we came home and my mom was passed out on the couch. I didn't understand that she was drunk; I thought she was just taking a nap. She woke up later, didn't remember us ever coming home from school. Rip-roaring drunk, she came and found us on the playground and proceeded to beat me up. Someone called the police on her. It was a huge trauma.*
>
> *"I really think this was because of the demon she was living with and that was the only way she could cope. The prior generations were a lot less likely to explore treatment. Had she been in therapy and maybe getting the kind of help she needed, her life could have been happier, and also my sister's life and my own."*

A number of the parents I spoke to said it was precisely this kind of memory that motivated them to seek help for their children. They simply did not want to let family history repeat itself. "Juliette," a respondent to my "Second Thoughts" column in the *Times*, provided another example:

> *"I was a naysayer until faced with a child who, at age seven, still could not reliably spell her own first name correctly, despite being in the gifted range in verbal IQ. We, too, tried a laundry list of alternative dietary, behavioral, and medical treatments before resorting to stimulant meds and an intensive-reading program for dyslexics. The result: a second-grader who has progressed from a kindergarten to a fourth-grade reading level in a matter of months. She is even more thrilled than we are. It's hard to express what this first taste of success means to a child who has felt like a failure her whole life.*
>
> *"For those who feel there's been an increase in kids with 'issues' in recent years, or attribute parents' decision to medicate to an overemphasis on having 'high-achieving' kids, I think the case of my own father, who's now seventy-six, is instructive. When he was a child, he had a profile almost identical to that of my daughter. He just didn't get anything. He was completely hopeless in school. His teachers knew he was bright, and the only label they had to make sense of his difficulties was 'lazy.' He dropped out of school and—despite the fact that he eventually pulled it together and graduated from college, at the age of forty—became a lifelong alcoholic, prone to severe depression and panic attacks. When my daughter's ADHD was diagnosed, the writing was on the wall. We weren't going to let her end up like my dad."*

If you were reading newspapers over the past couple of years, you could easily have come away with the sense that ADHD is little more than a problem of immaturity, easily outgrown and of no lasting effect. But that just isn't true. The prognosis for untreated ADHD is actually quite grim.

For the disorder is not, contrary to much popular opinion, a benign, quasi-imaginary disorder that goes away when kids grow up and "learn to behave." It's actually, recent research shows, a disorder of brain maturation, with wide-ranging effects on children's abilities to think, reason, learn, socialize, and otherwise develop like their peers. Children with ADHD go through life with brains that are basically three to five years behind those of other kids their age. And while their brains' physical development eventually catches up, the long-term effects of all those years of delay do not just go away. The reason, explains John March, a professor of psychiatry and chief of child and adolescent psychiatry at Duke University Medical Center, is that "it's bad for the brain to be mentally ill. The brain grows by learning," he told me. "If you're mentally ill, what your brain learns is mental illness. If you reduce the symptoms of mental illness, the bet is that the brain will learn to be more normal."

Fully two-thirds of children with ADHD carry symptoms of the disorder forward into adulthood, Philip Shaw, a psychiatrist at the National Institute of Mental Health and lead author of the groundbreaking brain-imaging study that in late 2007 showed the structural differences and developmental delays in the brains of children with ADHD, told me. Adults with ADHD aren't hyper, but they're inattentive, have difficulty staying on task, very often have other mental health disorders and, at the very least, bear the baggage of their childhood travails, which can translate into a greatly impaired sense of competency and greatly reduced self-esteem. "It's really a partial remission," he said. "And it's really impairing for people."

Untreated children with ADHD are 32 to 40 percent more likely than others to drop out of school and have significant difficulties completing college, 50 to 70 percent more likely to have few or no friends, 70 to 80 percent more likely to underperform at work when they grow up, and 40 to 50 percent more likely to engage in antisocial behavior and to use tobacco or illicit drugs. Children growing up with ADHD are 40 percent more likely to experience teen pregnancy, to speed and have car accidents, 20 to 30 percent more likely to experience depression as adults, "and in hundreds of other ways mismanage and endanger their lives," the authors of an "International Consensus Statement on ADHD," published in the *Clinical Child and Family Psychology Review*, wrote in 2002.

Prognoses for kids who don't get services for autism are, as one might expect, even worse. Without top-quality interventions, 45 percent of autistic children will require extensive government support, including institutionalization and round-the-clock care as they age. Another 45 percent will need at least some public support, such as work programs, living assistance, and Medicaid. But if they receive proper treatment and intervention, only 10 percent will require extensive government aid, 55 percent will need some assistance, and 35 percent (as opposed to 10 percent) will be able to live independently without support.

March's formulation—that it's "bad for the brain" to be mentally ill, holds up for autism as well as ADHD. And, of course, it holds up for other mental disorders as well.

Children with untreated minor depression are at risk for much more serious episodes of major depression later in life, some research psychiatrists now believe. The reason, they say, is that depression is essentially toxic for the developing brain, a form of stress that makes the brain more prone to later and worse depression. "If you get depressed as a child or adolescent, it changes the brain. It scars the brain," William Stixrud, a prominent Washington, D.C., area neuropsychologist, who serves on the faculty of both the George Washington University Medical Center and the Division of Child and Adolescent Psychiatry at Georgetown University Medical School, informed me. Childhood anxiety disorders, too, are now believed to prime the brain for later episodes of depression, if they go untreated. "What we've got to do is prevent depression," Stixrud said. "And you prevent depression in part by treating anxiety disorders, because anxiety disorders are your best prediction if you're going to get depressed."

The Connecticut mother I mentioned before saw firsthand what can happen if a child's mental health disorder goes too long untreated. Her daughter began to have serious mood problems in seventh grade and went into therapy. But it was three years before she was diagnosed with bipolar disorder and put on appropriate medication. By the time this happened, she was in such bad shape that she couldn't function in school. She had to drop out and be homeschooled for the remainder of that year.

"If someone is underdiagnosed and it's a severe case," her mother told me, "their life is basically thrown away."

All the focus in our public debate has been on the overtreatment, the overdiagnosing, the overmedicating of children, and the parental perfidy that allegedly accompanies it. But what of parents' responsibility to take the best possible care of their kids, using the best resources and services available to them? Our society pursues parents who choose to deny their children needed medical care in courts of law. Why do we castigate those who provide their children with needed psychiatric care?

I wonder if it's time for parents who do so to come out of their defensive crouch and stand up for what is, in fact, a moral choice. As Harold Koplewicz put it in his 1996 book, *It's Nobody's Fault,* when a child is showing symptoms of a mental disorder, "finding the right treatment is a parent's responsibility. Parents don't make their children sick, but it is their job to do everything possible to see that their kids get better."

At the very least, they can do what they can to insure that their kids don't grow up to be adults who make their own children miserable.

• • •

There are all kinds of statistics available on children's mental health diagnoses and psychotropic drug use. But—as was the case with the Valium numbers in the 1970s—the story they tell isn't clear. You can see how many scripts have been written or filled—but you don't know if the pills were ever used. (Or how much time they covered; a prescription for stimulants, for example, cannot be refilled, as stimulants are controlled substances. This then requires many prescriptions to be written for one person over the course of a year.) You can see the numbers of diagnoses given—but you don't know if they were true or false, too liberally or too conservatively made. We don't know the quality or the caliber of the conversations taking place in the offices of child psychiatrists, psychologists, and pediatricians. We don't have any way to quantify the degree of suffering reflected by the prescription or diagnosis or the office visit numbers. So, in the end, we can spin those numbers to tell virtually any story we want them to tell.

The dominant story these days is that of the overdiagnosed and overmedicated child and his or her lazy, competitive parent.

I'm going to argue now, however, that other stories are possible.

There is a story of progress—that children finally are being treated for problems that in the past they would have had to suffer through without recognition or care.

There is a story of missed opportunity—that too many children aren't getting the considerable help that now could be offered to them.

And there is the story of wasted opportunity and progress betrayed: how psychiatrists, the drug companies, and others involved in the business of providing services to children have, through offensive business practices, questionable relationships, arrogance, insouciance, and, at times, out-and-out quackery, lost the public trust, squandering the promise of the moment.

These alternative narratives, I believe, combined into one mixed and nuanced story, form an accurate account of what's happening in the area of children's mental health in our time. We need to shift our thinking away from the story line of b-a-d children and worse parents and toward this new message, not only because it is true, but also, quite simply, because it does no harm and, in addition, has the potential to lead in the direction of a great deal of good.

In this chapter, I shared stories of stigma. Now I want to move on to stories of progress—and of progress betrayed.

· 10 ·

A "Better Time Than Ever"

"Just thirty years ago, my daughter Isabel might have been labeled mentally retarded, and there would have been little opportunity for her to find her place in the world," Roy Richard Grinker writes in the introduction to his 2007 book, *Unstrange Minds: Remapping the World of Autism*, which begins with an account of how he and his wife struggled to get help for their daughter, Isabel, who was born in 1991, and diagnosed as autistic in 1994. "Our family," he continues, "would have been at a loss as to what to do.

> *"Isabel would probably have been placed in a residential institution with a minimal education plan, where the symptoms of her autism would have worsened. A mildly autistic child living at the same time at home would have been teased and bullied mercilessly, would have had little access to special-education services, and would have failed at school and suffered profound emotional distress. Pediatricians, mental health care practitioners, speech and occupational therapists, and educators still need to know more about autism, but they know enough now to make a big difference. They are diagnosing autism and providing therapy to children with autism at earlier ages than ever, and they are dis-*

> *covering how to use safe and effective medicines to ameliorate some of the symptoms of autism. Now my teenage daughter is mainstreamed into a high school classroom for part of the day. Numerous tests have shown that she has above average intelligence. She even plays cello in the school orchestra.*

"Autism is a terrible, lifelong disorder," he concludes, "but it's a better time than ever to be autistic."

As we've seen, parents of children with mental health issues, and the doctors who treat those children, tend to see the drama of the diagnosed and "medicated" child in our time in a way that's very different from received wisdom.

Where the general public sees overdiagnosis, they see much-needed help. Where the public sees overmedication, they see, at worst, a necessary evil, and, in many cases, a godsend. Where we tend to worry, as a culture, about the destruction of childhood, they see the opening-up of childhood's challenges and pleasures to kids who, in the past, wouldn't ever have had a chance to experience them.

When you take this perspective into account; that is to say, place the experience of the mentally ill child at the center, rather than the sidelines of the debate, then the developments of the past few decades become a story of progress.

For, the fact is that understanding mental disorders as brain dysfunction rather than as a breakdown of mothering have led to treatments that actually allow children to improve and live their lives to the fullest. Now that the "parentectomy"—excision of parental influence—is no longer the cornerstone of treatment, as it was, in particular, for autism in the past, children are no longer put in mental hospitals for years at a time, dropping out of school and home life, and severing all connection to the everyday world, in order to undergo intensive, and sometimes heavily tranquilized, psychoanalysis. (Joanne Greenberg's psychoanalytic mental hospital, brought to life in *I Never Promised You a Rose Garden*, was, even in its day, an anomaly in its total refusal to treat patients with psychotropic drugs. Mindy Lewis's Thorazine-fogged two and a half years at Columbia-Presbyterian was a more typical experience.)

Anorexics stay home and learn to eat again with the support of their families. Children with mental health disorders go to school. They go to camp. They go to college.

Their medications—in the much-commented-upon camp "med lines"—shock sensibilities. Their needs sometimes overwhelm college mental health services. And yet, their very presence at school, camp, and college tells another story: that there are treatments for kids today that, on the whole, *actually work.*

Twenty years of scientific research (funded, in the early years, largely without drug company money) has shown that antidepressant medication, when coupled with cognitive behavioral therapy, works for 60 to 80 percent of children suffering from depression and anxiety disorders. (There are, of course, a number of highly publicized studies that show that antidepressants don't work at all; that they're no more effective than placebo. I have heard two explanations for this from doctors who do believe they work—at least for some people. One is that the negative results stemmed from drug company studies where subjects were undermedicated, given such low doses of medication, in order to minimize the chance of side effects, that a therapeutic dose was never reached. Another is that what such studies have shown is *not* that the antidepressants didn't work, but that the placebo effect was disproportionately huge because the studies were very poorly designed and hastily conducted, with an eye to getting drugs to market as quickly as possible.)

Research has shown stimulant medications to be effective for 70 to 80 percent of kids with ADHD. And those who get some behavioral therapy in addition do even better.

"In fact," Dr. Darshak Sanghavi, chief of pediatric cardiology and an assistant professor of pediatrics at the University of Massachusetts Medical School, wrote in a piece headlined "Ritalin Fears Overblown" that ran in *The Boston Globe* in 2005, "the increased diagnosis and treatment of ADHD may be a major public health success story."

There are a lot of success stories.

Children considered all but untreatable a generation ago now have doctors who talk about "cures." Children with obsessive-compulsive disorder, for example, considered hopeless cases in just the mid-1980s, are now helped enormously by cognitive behavioral therapy, either alone or with medication. Vast numbers of children formerly called "mentally retarded" are now diagnosed as autistic and can be helped, with specialized therapies that can teach many of them to communicate and connect.

Children with learning disabilities can be tutored so skillfully and specifically that they can learn to function—and thrive—in the educational mainstream. With the right kind of specialized, intensive tutoring, children with dyslexia can actually have their brains changed so that new, compensatory neurocircuits are created to replace circuits that aren't functioning normally. One 2007 report out of Oregon, which showed the demand for the state's special-education services to be greatly on the rise, also indicated that the biggest group of children traditionally put in special ed—those with learning disabilities—was shrinking, because early intervention programs were catching children's learning issues at a much younger age and were remedying them so well that the children did not have to stay in special education later.

It's the shift away from parent-bashing, "from the era of blame and shame where children were always the victims and parents were always the villains," that has made all this progress possible, NIMH director Thomas Insel told me in 2009. "Understanding all these disorders—schizophrenia, autism, ADHD, bipolar disorder, mood and anxiety disorders—everything the NIMH does [learning disability research, too]—as developmental brain disorders, problems of the way brain circuits are getting laid down," he said, "is a fundamental shift. It's revolutionary."

The dyslexia model—in which brain retraining "therapy" has actually proven itself capable of rewiring the cortex—is the goal now of all child psychiatry, Insel said. Or it should be. And it can be, he said, thanks to the emergence very recently of new tools to study brain circuitry, and the growth of interest in, and funding for, the burgeoning new field of developmental neuroscience.

Developmental neuroscience, an interdisciplinary area of study drawing together genetics, neuroscience, physiology, developmental psychology, and epidemiology, hasn't really seeped into popular awareness so far. But it's the future of child psychiatry, which is to say, it's the future of all psychiatry, Duke University psychiatrist John March, who cochaired a workgroup for the NIMH on neurodevelopmental research in 2007, told me, because all the current research is indicating that, if you want to treat, prevent, even hope to "cure" mental illness, you've got to start with kids.

"Child psychiatry will really be the heart of psychiatry in the future," March said, in February 2009. "Epidemiology now shows that if you're mentally ill as an adult, you first were mentally ill as a child or an adolescent. This shows we have to stop thinking about mentally ill children as an afterthought to mental illness in adults: the horse is out of the barn by adulthood. In people with the gene that puts them at risk for Alzheimer's you can see brain differences show up in teenagers—but the disease doesn't show up for another fifty years. Many if not most of these gene variants now being identified as vulnerability factors for mental illness—and this is true for schizophrenia, mood and anxiety disorders, autism, and all the rest—actually are active in early brain development. They're part of the processes by which neurons go where they're supposed to go and find adjacent neurons and set up proper conversations."

That process "breaks down" in the brains of people who are developing disorders like schizophrenia and autism, March said. "The neurons don't migrate properly or in some cases they don't set up functional conversations when and where they're supposed to."

The work of developmental neuroscience is to look at the brain's plasticity, see how things go wrong in development, and figure out what kinds of interventions can correct what's going wrong, either to make the brain function normally or to compensate for what's not functioning normally, and ultimately to get the brain to start functioning differently.

Doing this, Insel clarified, will ultimately mean having to redefine what mental illness is. Right now, via the *DSM-IV*, we identify disorders by their symptoms—attention deficits, anxiety, depression, for example; eventually, he said, we'll identify them by their biological cause. "Attention-deficit/hyperactivity disorder—think about that," he said. "It's as though I said people with ischemic heart disease had a disorder of chest pain." Ultimately, he said, the goal will be to learn to recognize the very earliest signs that something developmental is going awry, and then to intervene as soon as possible, even before symptoms of mental illness start to show up.

"The behavioral and cognitive manifestations you see with mental illnesses are the tip of the iceberg," Insel said.

"No," he corrected himself. "That's the wrong metaphor.

> *"They're the end stage of disease, the heart attack after many, many things have been going on for some time. Cardiology only moved forward when it was established that heart attack is a late stage of disease. For the past one hundred years, we've been defining schizophrenia by the presence of psychosis. I'm suggesting this is a developmental disorder; if someone has a psychotic break, it's the end stage of the disease. If you want to move forward, you have to treat preventively. If we were really smart, we'd have biomarkers and predictors and know who's really at risk and intervene long before you had these cognitive and behavioral difficulties and realize that the interventions are not the same as they*

> *are for the end stage of the disorders. With cardiology it's diet and exercise and statins—that's different from the end-stage interventions after someone has a heart attack. We don't know yet what the statin-intervention would be for someone with bipolar disorder or autism or OCD."*

Schizophrenia researchers are already trying to figure out whether an earlier, incomplete form of the illness—they call it a "schizophrenia prodrome"—exists in kids, and if so, how to treat it. Some researchers have begun treating very disturbed but not quite psychotic teens with antipsychotic medications and cognitive behavioral therapy to see if they can keep them from developing the full-blown illness as adults or, at least, delay the expected onset of their symptoms. (To date, the results are very mixed, and the risks, from antipsychotic medications, at least, very high.)

There is preliminary work along those lines also being done with children who appear to have mini-episodes of bipolar disorder—very short episodes of dramatic mood swings—to see if treating such children could prevent them from developing a full-blown version of the disorder. Another line of neurodevelopmental research with suspected bipolar kids has another goal entirely: to try to greatly reduce false diagnoses of pediatric bipolar disorder by figuring out exactly what differentiates the brains of kids who truly have the disorder from those who don't.

That research is extremely preliminary, too, though at least one brain imaging study has indicated that bipolar kids show some brain anomalies that indicate specific deficits in cognition and in how they process emotions, Ellen Leibenluft, chief of the Section on Bipolar Spectrum Disorders in the Emotion and Development Branch of the Mood and Anxiety Disorders Program at the National Institute of Mental Health, told me.

If these differences hold up in future research, or if other such biomarkers are found and can be put to use in making diagnoses, she believes, it would be an invaluable advance in the proper treatment of the many kids who are today being lumped together as bipolar. This could lead to a real reduction in the use of powerful antipsychotic medications. It could also, Leibenluft said, potentially help in identifying true bipolar children much earlier; early enough, in fact, that they could perhaps be treated with nondrug interventions, and be kept from developing the full-blown symptoms that land them on medication. These interventions could include structured psychotherapy to help kids learn to regulate their emotions and control their behavior, or cognitive behavioral techniques for depression. Family therapy has proven useful too in helping parents deal more constructively with bipolar children in treatment, she said.

This was the great surprise I had in learning about this most recent research effort in biological psychiatry: While the goal of the scientists involved in it was biological change—of the brain and its circuitry—they didn't necessarily equate that change with "better living through chemistry." Instead, what came up, over and over again, was therapy—particularly cognitive behavioral therapy—either as an adjunct to or, when possible, a replacement for, medication.

Which isn't to say that the doctors were medication-averse. On the contrary, there have been research discoveries in recent years that, many say, may indicate that a whole new era in pharmacotherapy could be beginning. The great model for this is the very recent discoveries regarding Fragile X Syndrome, a genetic condition that can cause learning disabilities, severe mental impairment, and autism.

Scientists have now identified both the specific genetic mutation that causes Fragile X Syndrome and what that mutation does, which is to knock out one of the brakes on fast-acting excitatory neurotransmission in the brain. While the protein cannot be repaired, the right kind of drug can intervene in the neuronal processes that are going awry, so that brain cells begin to act normally. Fragile X mice, treated in this way, no longer show signs of abnormality. Human studies are just beginning.

Very recent brain imaging studies in kids with ADHD seem to indicate that stimulant medications *may* also restore normal neurodevelopment processes: that is to say, make kids' developmentally delayed brains look normal. As I mentioned, recent studies indicate that the brains of children with ADHD show a three- to five-year developmental lag behind those of children without the disorder. With medication, these children's brains can actually look normal. "The twelve-year-old with ADHD looks like a nine-year-old without," Insel explained. "The most recent data shows the psychostimulants actually accelerate cortical maturation so that they normalize."

Some researchers now say that antidepressants may not only lessen symptoms of depression but actually could promote brain resilience, helping protect the brain against the ravages of depression and future episodes. The hope, in the future, is to develop drugs that could specifically help shield the brain against the effects of stress hormones, based on the theory that people with depression are particularly susceptible to the toxic effects of stress.

"The bet we are placing in the lives of American kids is that the medications are neuroprotective . . . that they address particular molecular mechanisms that reflect the underlying neurobiology of the illness; they don't just address symptoms," March told me. "If medications can help the mentally ill child learn and develop more normally, the bet is that the brain will learn to be more normal."

In the same way, he continued, cognitive behavioral therapy teaches the brain to be "more normal," by directly working on skills that are not developing as they should be, because mental illness is getting in the way.

"CBT targets specific brain processes that are tied to specific behaviors," he said. "It's analogous to medical care. With mental illness, a CBT therapist targets learning mechanisms that either rehabilitate the affected circuitry or develop compensatory circuitry like with dyslexia, which takes over for the circuitry that's not working."

That's why, March said, kids with mood and anxiety disorders who get treated with cognitive behavioral therapy in combination with medication can do so incredibly well—even "normalize"—in a matter of months.

That is to say, if they get that kind of care. Which they very rarely do.

"The best of what we know how to do can be very good," he said. But he added, "Unless you are lucky enough to find your way to a specialized medical setting, if you're a mentally ill kid, you don't have a chance in hell of getting that kind of care."

This is the irony and the tragedy of our Brave New World of children's mental health care: At a time when we have treatments that actually work, when there's more research than ever before, more knowledge, better understanding, more support in the schools, and more public awareness of the dangers of untreated mental illness, the actual caretaking that kids with mental health needs receive is, for the most part, really poor.

In Chapter 3, I discussed the fact that most children with mental health issues get no care at all. Those who do get care most of the time receive services that come nowhere close to what is accepted as the best standard of practice within the mental health field.

As I mentioned earlier, in the past couple of years, there's been considerable attention given to the fact that foster children are being treated with surprisingly high levels of psychotropic medication, aren't being monitored properly during their use, and, as a number of state attorneys general have charged, are essentially being used as state-funded guinea pigs in pharmaceutical company-promoted experiments in off-label drug use. But it isn't just foster kids, children in the child welfare system, and children on Medicaid—our country's poorest and most vulnerable—who aren't getting decent care.

The lack of good care in our country is epidemic.

In a series of studies published in 2005, the National Institute of Mental Health found that only a third of the treatments people were receiving across the country for their mental disorders met minimal standards of effectiveness. Things are no better for children.

For one thing, they're not seeing specialists. Most children with mental health issues get their care—if they get any—from pediatricians. And pediatricians can't do anything even approaching a thorough diagnosis in the eight to twelve minutes that, on average, insurance restrictions permit them to spend with patients. Most, as I mentioned earlier, don't want to bear the responsibility for treating children with mental health issues. And yet many have no choice, if their patients live in an underserved area or if the parents of their patients can't afford to pay for mental health care.

Even when children are referred out for specialty care, most do not receive very good care. Although a number of government studies have now established that children who receive some combination of medication and therapy—generally, cognitive behavioral therapy—have the best outcomes, few actually receive that kind of comprehensive treatment. In part, the problem is that real life rarely offers the kind of access to top-flight care that children who participate in research studies receive.

This message emerged very strongly from the most extensive study on ADHD treatment to date, the National Institute of Mental Health's Collaborative Multisite Multimodal Treatment Study of Children with ADHD, or MTA study, which was published in 1999. The MTA study brought together eighteen leading researchers in ADHD at six different university medical centers and hospitals, and included nearly six-hundred children aged seven to nine, who were divided into groups receiving medication only, medication plus behavioral therapy, behavioral therapy alone, and routine community care, and followed for an initial period of fourteen months, with follow-up studies published in 2004 and 2007. It found that two-thirds of children with ADHD who received top-notch care—a mixture of carefully controlled stimulant medication and behavioral therapy—improved so much that their behavior actually became "normal."

But most kids never get that level of treatment. In the MTA study, kids who were in the "community care" group—i.e. receiving treatment from regular doctors in their home communities, at a level of care typical of what most kids around the country get if they've been diagnosed with ADHD—got nothing like it at all. Two-thirds of the kids in the "community" group were given medication, and about a fourth got some kind of therapy. But they only saw their pediatricians about twice a year, and the handling of the medication was "pretty haphazard," Peter Jensen, the former associate director of child and adolescent research at the NIMH and the lead author of a 2007 three-year follow-up of the MTA study, told me.

On the other hand, the kids in the MTA researchers' "medication" group, or "medication plus therapy" group, got a half-hour visit with a pediatrician once a month. The pediatrician also met with the child's family one half-hour per month, and collected behavior rating scales from both teachers and parents—a degree of close follow-up with school personnel that, other researchers have found, only a "small proportion" of doctors ever do.

The kids getting behavioral therapy, either alone or with medication, were treated using carefully developed behavioral protocols for ADHD devised by William E. Pelham Jr., a psychologist at SUNY–Buffalo. All this close monitoring and follow-up, particularly when coupled with highly specialized behavioral therapy, led to incredible results. The medication groups did *twice* as well as the community group. Kids who got medication plus specialized behavior therapy had the most spectacular results of all. "It even affected how well kids were liked by other kids," Jensen said.

Comprehensive care, follow-up, close monitoring, treating a child in the larger context of school and family, really matters. Because medication, even when highly effective, can't do it all. This message came through very clearly in parent responses to the MTA study, as recorded by researchers in a 2004 follow-up article. The researchers noted, with some surprise, that, although medication alone or medication plus therapy was by far most effective in reducing ADHD core symptoms (things like inattention and impulsivity), parents were most satisfied when children didn't get meds, but got behavioral therapy instead. Symptom-wise, these children didn't improve anywhere nearly as much as the kids who got medication, but they did learn, via therapy, to get along better with their parents, an essential improvement, coupled, undoubtedly, with the psychological plus of avoiding medication, that made everyone happier.

Kids with mental health issues in America today generally don't get treatments that take time and don't get treatments that cost a lot of money, both of which comprehensive care always does. It doesn't seem to matter how many government studies prove the importance of combining medication with evidence-based therapy, or how many news reports drive home the dangers of medication.

What's driving the mental health care of kids today is the bottom line: cost control measures decided upon by health insurance companies. And that means that, instead of comprehensive care, kids just get medication. All too often, kids end up on multiple medications, even though there's no solid scientific evidence to back the practice. Children end up multiply medicated because they have multiple symptoms, because their primary medications produce multiple side effects, and because all those symptoms and all those side effects just can't be addressed in a reimbursable, fifteen-minute med-check visit.

The multiple use of medications, many child psychiatrists agree, is one of the worst developments to have come out of the managed care–driven health system we have today. Also destructive is the way money pressures have fractured the delivery of mental health care, turning psychiatrists into quick-visit medicine givers, and shifting the practice of therapy almost exclusively over to psychologists and, increasingly, much less expensive (and less extensively trained) social workers.

Psychiatrists, pediatricians, and psychotherapists should coordinate care, but they don't necessarily do it. They also don't necessarily speak the same conceptual language. There's great insularity within the professions, beginning in medical schools, where psychologists and psychiatrists are trained separately and often taught to think of each other as antagonists. So cognitive behavioral therapy, for example, remains the almost exclusive province of psychologists. And psychiatrists are putting up a strong front of resistance against the growing number of psychologists who want to be able to be trained and licensed to prescribe medication. And, of course, the quality of mental health practitioners, at all levels of the food chain, varies so very greatly.

"Children treated skillfully are helped," March said. "Those who don't receive evidence-based quality care not only are not likely to be helped but may in fact be damaged."

Great help for children with mental health issues exists. And yet, science has far outpaced our capacity to use it well. Progress has been betrayed by commercial interests, political complaisance, and a lack of policy directed at making sure that new scientific advances are safely and with oversight made available to and accessible for the public.

This could be fixed. There should be gatekeepers within our health care system shepherding parents toward getting the best treatments. There should be protocols for what these best treatments consist of. There should be safeguards against profiteering and quackery. There should be affordable access. There should be guidance, and protections in place to make parents feel that they can trust that whatever care their children receive is safe, necessary, and of proven efficacy.

None of this is happening.

Instead, there is nontreatment and sloppily administered drug treatment. There are therapies and interventions on the market of dubious value. There are entrepreneurs selling extremely expensive brain scans that they claim can "show" the existence of mental disorders, and which brain researchers uniformly say are interesting, even pretty, but of no actual value in diagnosis or treatment. There are optometrists claiming they can "cure" ADHD, learning issues, and dyslexia through eye exercises, even though the American Academy of Pediatrics, among other doctors' groups, has repeatedly declared that vision problems are not the primary cause of learning disabilities and that vision therapy is a waste of time and money. ("Ineffective, controversial methods of treatment such as vision therapy may give parents and teachers a false sense of security that a child's learning difficulties are being addressed, may waste family and/or school resources, and may delay proper instruction or remediation," is how the latest statement from the Academy put it, in July 2009.)

There are virtually no guidelines, no gatekeepers—other than the insurance companies, who essentially create protocols for care according to what they will pay for. The net result is that parents feel they're all alone, navigating an all but nonexistent child mental health care system—"a little like Hansel and Gretel going into the dark forest, trying to mark your bearings with bread crumbs," as the mother of a boy with ADHD put it to me.

Journalist Paul Raeburn's account of his struggles to secure good, consistent care for his bipolar son and severely depressed daughter, recounted in his book, *Acquainted with the Night*, captures the situation:

> *"We needed help from someone. But when we tried to find it, it wasn't there. We took the children to a series of psychiatrists who repeatedly misdiagnosed them and treated them incorrectly, sometimes making them worse. We talked to therapists who threw us off course again and again with faulty assessments. We took the children to hospitals that did not keep them long enough to help them, because our insurance company wouldn't pay for the care. We talked to school officials who must have seen dozens or hundreds of troubled kids, but who told us they'd never seen such problems before and had no idea what to do. We spent tens of thousands of dollars, some of the money wasted on inappropriate care, to try to fill the vast gaps in our insurance plan. Sometimes these efforts helped, sometimes they didn't.*
>
> *"What we found was a splintered, chaotic mental health care system that seemed to do more harm than good."*

The parents I interviewed for this book were mostly people who should have had access to good care. They were middle- and upper-middle-class; they were employed; most lived in big cities where there were a lot of providers. And yet they told me stories, time and again, of poor care.

There were stories of unprofessional behavior: One South Carolina doctor, consulted by a mother and father to help deal with their son's anxiety and learning issues, concentrated instead on trying to convert the dad, who is Muslim, to Christianity.

There were stories of just-plain-weird therapy: "Take the one thing she really loves and when she doesn't obey take it to Goodwill and give it away," an adoption therapist told one California mother, whose adopted three-year-old from a Russian orphanage was biting, spitting, throwing tantrums, and "revenge peeing" in anger. When the mother protested that this sounded cruel, the therapist responded, "'Do you want to wind up with a Mother Teresa or a Hitler?'" the mother told me.

And, most commonly, there were stories of false starts, fragmented care, and practitioners of greatly varying talents, all of which meant that the process of getting help was a long, incredibly expensive one, with a lot of wrong turns and time wasted.

The Connecticut mother with the bipolar daughter went to the school guidance counselor when her daughter first started having symptoms in middle school. The guidance counselor recommended a family therapist. "[The therapist] said she was 'fine,' just had 'some issues,'" the mom told me.

The therapist brought the parents in for family sessions. He prided himself upon his holistic approach. He prescribed St. John's Wort, an herb commonly believed to have antidepressant properties. It made the girl "really hyper," the mom said.

> *"Finally, one day in ninth grade, she had this meltdown. In a store, she got really angry. She said, 'I'm going to hurt myself.' We took her to the hospital. They put her in a crisis center. They said nothing could be done; they didn't know what was wrong. They blamed me for being too overprotective. I decided to take her to a child psychiatrist. But all the child psychiatrists I called had five-month waits for appointments. I called the pediatrician, who knew a good psychiatrist who owed her a favor. We got an appointment a month later.*

"The psychiatrist diagnosed her on the spot," the mother told me.

> *"She said, 'She's rapid cycling before my eyes.' I realized that she'd been rapid cycling ten to twelve times a day. I didn't know what it was. She'd be very happy and funny one second, very sad the next. I'd just thought it was normal teen angst.*

"The psychiatrist prescribed medication. I called the family therapist.

"'Didn't you see anything?' I asked him.

"He said that, when the St. John's Wort had made her hyper, he'd suspected that she might be bipolar. He said he was hoping to treat it another way. I think he just didn't want to lose the patient. He had us going to family therapy, milking the whole thing, making us come in and pay for a session whenever we had a question. Never once did he mention the diagnosis."

Having access to the "best" doctors, however, is no guarantee that a family will find good care.

The greater Washington, D.C., area, home to Children's National Medical Center, the National Institute of Mental Health, and the medical schools of George Washington University, Georgetown, and Johns Hopkins, plus a lot of well-off parents, has no shortage of child specialists. Some of the country's top names in the treatment of autism, anxiety disorders, ADHD, and other mental health problems are clustered there. And yet, local parents' odysseys in finding good care for their children were no shorter, or less circuitous, than those of parents in other parts of the country. I heard repeatedly of well-thought-of pediatricians who pooh-poohed mothers' concerns and of much-solicited mental health specialists who repaid parents' willingness to pony up steep fees with inexcusable arrogance.

One D.C. mom told me of taking her eight-year-old daughter to a psychologist for the first time. The psychologist started the intake session thirty minutes late and, then, ten minutes later, called the parents in for a discussion.

"She said, 'I did some Rorschach testing,'" the mother told me. "'I only had to show three inkblots. She saw a bug. This shows people who can't share their hearts.' She diagnosed my daughter as 'fundamentally depressed.'"

When the parents pressed the psychologist to explain further, she refused—there were only ten minutes left in the session, she said. But she did recommend that the girl begin vision therapy. She'd noted that she had some problems with block assembly.

"I never experienced something so unprofessional and so irresponsible," the mother told me, irate.

Another local mother called a psychiatrist to make an appointment for her difficult daughter and was told, after a brief conversation by phone, that the little girl was "probably bipolar." A week of agony for the mother ensued, ending with an office appointment in which the psychiatrist said the girl wasn't bipolar at all. She had ADHD.

The mother demanded an explanation.

"Sorry," the psychiatrist said. "They were doing construction outside my window on the day you called. I guess I got a little distracted."

One well-known doctor, a national name in autism treatment, charged the parents of a young boy $700 for an intake consultation. "It was just awful," the mother told me. "We were sitting in his house and were kept waiting for forty-five minutes in an unheated area. He was eating and we thought he was taking notes, but really he was editing a paper. He kept leaving the room to reheat his lunch."

Treatment with another nationally renowned "name" doctor landed a seven-year-old boy, who was in treatment for ADHD but ultimately turned out to be bipolar, on the psychiatric ward of Children's Hospital in D.C. for two weeks. "His physician—the big specialist—had him on so much Tegretol that he'd lost the motor skills to pick up a fork, and on so much Prozac that he'd unleashed his bipolar disorder," the boy's mother said.

This was in the late 1990s, when the interactions between SSRIs and pediatric bipolar disorder were perhaps less well understood. The mother, a former clinical social worker, said it wasn't easy, in the early years, to untangle the problems plaguing her son, who was dyslexic, hyperactive, anxious, and often out of control, and that she believes the doctor was doing his best. She is less charitable, however, toward the social worker at Children's Hospital who, adding insult to injury at a moment of crisis, and with no prior knowledge of the family, took her and her husband to task for the obvious tensions in their marriage.

"At Children's the social worker said that everything that was wrong with our son was our fault," she said. "I knew enough as a social worker not to say anything like that even if you thought it was true. [The social worker's] idea was that we should have a romantic weekend away while my son was in the hospital. Never mind that I had this five-year-old at home freaking out. It was offensive what we went through as parents."

Being surrounded by specialists didn't stop another D.C. family from wandering in the dark forest, without a compass, as they tried to figure out how to help their son, who has Asperger's syndrome.

"When I started observing that something was wrong with my son, it was when he was opening and closing doors a lot and flipping light switches and not talking," the boy's mother told me. "He never babbled. He had a lot of ear infections as a child."

She and her husband went to consult a team of specialists. The doctors ran a battery of tests. They found nothing wrong with the boy. And yet, he was really very different from other children. He developed a habit of repeating back what other people said, reversing pronouns, repeating lines from movies and TV instead of making spontaneous conversation—like some autistic children do, the mother now knows. Yet, "autism never dawned on me," she said, looking back. "You don't know the right door to go into if you don't know what it is."

The boy's preschool said he had sensory integration dysfunction. It assigned two "shadows" to his classroom to follow him around during the day. The boy's pediatrician sent the mom to a developmental pediatric clinic at a local university hospital. "They suggested he get tested for a genetic disorder," the mom told me. "We got the report, which I laugh at to this day. It describes my son clearly with autistic behaviors—and then concludes that he's fine."

One doctor at the university hospital recommended that the boy be evaluated by a psychologist because he believed he was at risk for learning disabilities. The psychologist said she believed he was autistic, though he didn't meet all the criteria for the disorder. She diagnosed him with Pervasive Developmental Disorder-Not Otherwise Specified. "This was a good kick in the pants," the mom said. "We didn't know where to go next. [The psychologist] was new to the area and didn't know who to recommend us to go to. So we were all on our own."

The saga continued for another year. The boy began occupational therapy, tried a special diet and an auditory training program. One doctor recommended that he try vision therapy. Another said it wouldn't help and could be harmful.

He was tested again. He was said not to be autistic, just "an odd kid." Indeed, he got odder and odder, then, developing obsessions, becoming disruptive at school—and also teaching himself to read and scoring in the 99.6th percentile on intelligence tests. "You could give him any random date and he would know what day later in the year it would be," his mom said.

Finally, an educational consultant recommended that the family see a new doctor, a developmental and behavioral pediatrician. He did a full evaluation and a classroom observation and diagnosed the boy with Asperger's. Armed with a diagnosis that finally made sense, his parents were able to get him into a specialized private school. And, after a difficult year of transition, he began to thrive.

When I spoke to the mom, there were signs that her son had a bright future ahead of him. He was so high-functioning and was making such progress in school that, the developmental pediatrician said, a day might come when he would no longer even fit the criteria for Asperger's. While his mother was cautiously hopeful, she was still stunned by the length, expense, and plain weirdness of her family's mental health odyssey.

"We were sort of at the mercy of people," she said.

This is an impossible situation, and a cruel one, which transfers far too much of the burden of care and decision-making onto the backs of parents. And it is an unnecessary one.

In a country like ours, in a period like the present, there is absolutely no reason why children should be lacking for care or receiving substandard care. There is no reason why parents shouldn't be able to trust their doctors and the research upon which the doctors' decisions are made.

As I've said earlier, there have been real advances in child psychiatry in the past thirty years and there are some real success stories in treating ADHD, autism, OCD, dyslexia, and, arguably, in bringing down the teen suicide rate.

There are also some families who are able to access excellent care. I came across many success stories in the course of my research. Families who were able to feel truly taken care of and able to feel that their children were truly being helped.

These were families with money. And one extra piece of good fortune: a doctor—at least one—who took the time to truly get to know the child and his or her family, to think long and hard about that child's life and explore all options before embarking upon a course of treatment. It was that relationship that established trust. It was that relationship that helped work against false diagnoses and bad courses of medication. It was that relationship that helped parents work through stigma and helped children come to own their "issues" and play an active role in their own care.

Peter Jensen, who is now the president and CEO of the REACH Institute, a New York nonprofit aimed at disseminating the best information on children's mental health treatments to families and professionals, found this too, when he surveyed parents who'd undergone the odyssey of finding treatment for their children with ADHD. Eighty percent of the parents said that the one thing that had made the big difference in their quest was finding a doctor who gave them "love and support," Jensen told me.

"Doctors need to be fully aware of the complex human process of taking medicine," he said. "I call it the psychotherapy of pharmacotherapy. Parents have so many fears and worries. If you don't establish a good relationship, a warm, trusting relationship with the family, send love and support to the family, help with their grieving, help them to accept this child with all his or her difficulties . . . if as a doctor you just whip the pad out and say trust me, take this medicine, see you twice a year, that's when you see problems. Doctors have no business prescribing meds if they don't also establish a good relationship with the parents. If you do this, that love will be transmitted to the child."

Unfortunately, for most parents of children with mental health issues, feeling that love is a distant dream. The idea is almost laughable, really.

But it shouldn't have to be.

· 11 ·

Moving Forward

"I remember Richard. He was the disruptive kid thrown out of class—day after day after day—a class joke. I saw him recently at our fortieth high school reunion and asked him if he thought he had ADHD. He replied, 'Yes—and no one ever gave a damn.'"

JONANN, RESPONDING TO "SECOND THOUGHTS,"
NYTIMES.COM, MARCH 2, 2007

In the latter years of writing this book, I was haunted by two faces from my childhood. One face belonged to a family friend whom I'd known since nursery school. The other belonged to a member of my extended family.

Both boys—for the faces in my mind were of little boys—had been extremely smart and highly verbal children, what used to be called "precocious." The first boy had been funny and cute when he was very little. Teachers complained that his behavior wasn't great; he didn't work up to his potential; he spent a fair amount of time, as some boys did then, sitting on the floor out in the hall.

But as he grew older, he'd become kind of strange. He had a way of speaking that sounded rehearsed, as though he picked up words and phrases—even ways of thinking or feeling—from things he heard on TV. By high school, he was a mess. He pulled out all his eyebrows. He was a target for bullies. He went to college, but he couldn't finish. He never had a career, and his adult life never really got off the ground.

The other boy had been very clever. Funny. Always able to outsmart you in games. Always one step ahead of you in conversation. Always talking circles around you. And always in trouble.

He was always beating up his brother, breaking windows, getting in fights. He set a fire at his school once; his dad managed to talk the principal out of expelling him. He got away with things; he scraped by. It helped that he could do his schoolwork with his eyes closed.

The last I saw him, almost a decade ago, he was drunk, possibly stoned, and overflowing with a rage that made family members retreat from him in self-protection. I was later told by another relative that he was addicted to Valium.

Growing up, I'd never thought of these two boys as having had mental health issues. They were just, in the first instance, quirky, and in the second—well, everyone said he was bad.

But I thought of them almost incessantly once I became open to the idea that many of the children around us today who are labeled "weird" or "bad" actually have something going wrong with them. Something that can be addressed, interrupted, and, with hope, kept from wrecking their, and others', lives.

These boys came from families that were at the high end of the middle class. If they'd been in school today, they would most certainly have been "labeled" and diagnosed with something. (ADHD, ODD, anxiety, severe mood dysregulation?) My relative would almost certainly have been medicated.

And maybe, just maybe, his life would have been completely different.

Many of us have memories of the neighborhood oddball—often a brilliant child or teenager—who somehow went off the rails.

"From public school, you always remember the brilliant loser—the one who didn't integrate," mused the mother in Los Angeles who has struggled so mightily to reconcile her son's inattentive ADHD diagnosis with her beliefs about our *One Flew Over the Cuckoo's Nest* society, when we spoke, long and meanderingly, in the spring of 2007.

"There was a disconnect between who they were and what the world demanded," she said. "I remember one guy from school, he was very handsome and brilliant at math. He got into drugs. He ended up walking down Sunset Boulevard thinking he was Jesus Christ. He was really brilliant, but something didn't happen . . ."

She paused. Where, she wondered, was the line between a "free spirit" and a broken mind?

"Those were more permissive times," she finally sighed. "Maybe now, if he were more 'micromanaged,' he could have ended up a surgeon."

It so often looks like micromanaging, doesn't it—the testing, the labeling, the special interventions, the drugs for kids who are quirky, "weird," out-of-control, or sad?

How perverse it is that this is the spin we so instinctively give to parental behavior that is, at base, simply about making sure that, this time around at least, someone does "give a damn."

The fact that we think this way, that despite all the progress that's been made in understanding and treating kids' mental health disorders, we continue to talk in terms of bad kids and worse parents gaming the system, pushing for perfection, working every angle for their advantage, speaks volumes about where we are as a society today.

We are so anxious, so competitive, so worried about the future and our children's status, that we have shut down our hearts, shuttering much of our capacity for compassion. We are so rigid with anger, so judgmental in our insecurity. We are so profoundly distrustful, so sure of being cosmically ripped off.

We are terrified about "downward mobility," said historian Steven Mintz, when I called him in early 2008 to talk about the stories we tell about children in America today. Mintz is a specialist at dissecting how we weave narratives about children out of our own fears and worries and desires. His 2004 book, *Huck's Raft: A History of American Childhood,* highlighted a "pattern of recurrent moral panics over children's well being" starting in the early twentieth century, from fears of the emasculation of boys around 1910, to fears of juvenile delinquency in the 1950s, to fears of television in the early 1960s, fears of excessive child-centeredness in the late 1960s, to the familiar fears over teen pregnancy, stranger abductions, child abuse, drug use, and poor academic performance that skyrocketed in the 1970s and 1980s and persist among us, in the form of what he calls a "grossly inflated and misplaced sense of crisis" regarding kids today.

"Children have long served as a lightning rod for America's anxieties about society as a whole," he wrote.

> *"During the late 1940s and early 1950s, as anxiety about the Cold War deepened, many Americans doubted that the young had the moral fiber, intellectual acumen, and physical skills necessary to stand up to Communism. During the 1960s, as the nation underwent unsettling moral and cultural transformations, public worries again centered on the young, around such issues as permissive childrearing, youthful drug and sexual experimentation, and young people's scraggly hair and unkempt clothing. It is not surprising that cultural anxieties are often displaced on the young; unable to control the world around them, adults shift their attention to that which they think they can control: the next generation."*

As a society, we are now engaged in a similar sort of moral panic over the overdiagnosed, overmedicated child—the poster child for our competitive, Darwinian times. Society's alleged concern for him and others like him is a classic bit of displacement, containing all our fears of failure, downward mobility, and innocence lost, and largely unconcerned with the truth of mentally ill children's real challenges and needs.

We are so disgusted with parents and so disturbed by what we perceive to be the state of childhood today. And all that dislike, distrust, resentment, and fear have hardened our hearts. There is a nastiness, not just toward parents, but toward children, too, in the air.

Ginia Bellafante, the *New York Times* cultural critic, picked up on this in 2005, when she scanned the horizon of popular prime-time TV shows and sensed an insidious level of hostility toward children. (She returned to the topic, exploring "the literature of children in peril" in 2009.) Giving examples of a family therapist on *Criminal Minds* killing off the parents and children he treats in suburban Washington, a young mother on *ER* trying to kill herself and her children, and the fully half of *Law & Order: SVU* episodes over a six-year period that featured children as the "special victims," she observed that "child in peril" programming had replaced the "woman in peril" shows and films that began to fill the airwaves in the 1970s, signaling the beginning of the long backlash against feminism.

"Television has become an extremely inhospitable place for middle-class children, and in some sense, for the demanding ideals by which they are now raised—a gory receptacle for any and all of our collectively sublimated parental ambivalence," she wrote.

> *"Against our new universe of Humvee-inspired strollers, television constructs a parallel one, in which children are routinely maimed, killed, abused, mocked, mistreated and kept central. . . . Sometimes, actual harm is averted, but the message is always clear . . . children are trouble, make trouble, provoke trouble. . . .*
>
> *"But unspeakable acts of physical violence are just one part of the story. In the more realistic domain of shows specifically about family*

> *life, parents humiliate children, dismiss them, grow easily irritated by acts of childish self-expression, even though for much of recent memory, parents made every effort to woo their young as peers and friends, ensure their psychological maturity, spur them on to become confident and high achieving."*

More than twenty years now of exhausting, overbearing, competitive, anxious, narcissistic parenting have left a lot of people very angry. And rather than looking inward, many are displacing that anger outwards—onto today's children and other (it's always other) parents.

This, I believe, is at base the reason why the "love" that psychiatrist Peter Jensen mentioned at the end of the last chapter—writ large as the basis of comprehensive, compassionate care—isn't reaching the vast, vast majority of children with mental health issues.

These kids, and their parents, have been shut out in the cold.

It isn't just that the money isn't there to do right by their needs. There's a deficit of compassion, too.

When I began this book, I thought that the people involved in diagnosing and treating and thinking about and caring for children fell into two camps: there was the "humanistic" camp, which included anyone opposed to labeling or medicating kids, anyone who stood up for children's precious rights to be who they were and function as they functioned, and there were the biological psychiatrists, the enemies of free and natural human self-expression, who looked at children as symptom collections, and collaborated with high-strung parents who were willing to use any means necessary to prime their kids for ever-more-perfect performance.

But what I learned (when I actually learned something about the topic upon which I'd launched myself in ignorance) was that this way of viewing the subject was little less than ridiculous. I'd wandered into a turf war between different clans of children's mental health service providers, and I'd joined into a culture war—a battle medical historian Edward

Shorter has likened to "a religious war," without fully understanding the stakes or having an informed opinion of the players.

I know now that crying out against the "drugging" and pathologizing of children may seem very humanistic, a plea for human dignity and authenticity, but as a default response to the phenomenon of children's mental illness it isn't very humane. The truly humane response to sickness, to suffering, to distress, is to try to do something to make it go away.

If you really put children at the center of the debate about how we should treat their mental health issues, then there's really only one thing to say: They need to be helped to feel better. And their parents need to be helped to deal with them.

How do we do that? How do we as a society bring a kind of essential humanity to the treatment of kids with mental health issues? We have to start by advocating for better care.

In the last chapter, I mentioned that, among the dozens of people I interviewed, and the hundreds Peter Jensen reached in his research on parents of children with ADHD, the one thing that made an enormous difference in children's outcomes and family experiences, was the presence of one doctor who was able to take the time to get to know the child and his or her parents and truly listen to their concerns. This listening—this relationship—was the cornerstone of proper diagnosis and care that could change a child's life.

Health-care reform ought to make such time for listening an essential component of plans for the better delivery of care. Health insurance ought to pay for annual or semiannual extended visits with pediatricians to talk about children's lives and screen for mental health issues. Pediatricians should be made able to act as gatekeepers, to refer children out to mental health specialists if necessary, to consult with those specialists to coordinate treatment; in short, to act as a "medical home" for a child, as pediatrician John Stirling and child psychiatrist Lisa Amaya-Jackson put it in *Pediatrics* in 2008.

And then there need to be doctors for the pediatricians to refer parents to.

There need to be more child psychiatrists. Residency programs in child psychiatry can't even fill the relatively few slots they now have, Kristin Kroeger Ptakowski, senior deputy executive director and director of government affairs and clinical practice for the American Academy of Child and Adolescent Psychiatry told me. The field just isn't very appealing—it's low status within the practice of medicine, and, as medical specialties go, it's relatively low-paid. The training is long, and the expense for students is very great.

In recent years, legislation to address the workforce shortage—the Child Health Care Crisis Relief Act, which proposes providing loan forgiveness programs for child mental health professionals who agree to work in underserved areas—has languished in Congress. Perhaps this, too, might move forward with health care reform.

But even if many more child psychiatrists were to magically appear, as things now stand, most families couldn't afford for their children to see them in a way that would permit optimal care. Many child psychiatrists don't participate in health insurance.

And those child psychiatrists who do participate in health insurance aren't paid to do therapy, which means they can't provide the best standard of care recognized by their profession. It means that they are essentially boxed in to doing nothing more than medication management, solving each problem with pill after pill.

The shortsightedness of this approach has had its most dramatic impact on the country's sickest children with mental health issues who often end up in desperate straits, even in jail, because they don't get appropriate care within their communities. Structures simply don't exist now within communities to provide care at home for kids with very serious needs.

Wealthy parents can hire "shadows" to follow their kids at school and even keep things running smoothly at home—at personal costs that can run to thousands of dollars a week. But how many people can afford that kind of private, at-home care? Many kids with serious mental health issues end up getting care only after they've harmed themselves and ended up in the emergency room. (And even then, they slip through the cracks: One *Archives of General Psychiatry* report, in 2005, found "substantial under-recognition of mental illness" by emergency-room personnel, and showed that only half of the patients aged seven to twenty-four who were rushed to emergency rooms for self-inflicted injuries were assessed for possible mental health conditions.) Some, as I mentioned earlier, end up in the child welfare system, with the state footing the bill. It's a scandal that children's lives have to get *that bad* before they can receive help.

Are children without money essentially throwaway people? It seems that way sometimes in this country, never more than when you contemplate the inequities of our health care system. For children with mental health issues, a lack of care can truly lead to a life thrown away.

There have to be better incentives to get more child psychiatrists and psychologists to participate in health insurance. And reimbursement for psychiatrists who want to perform psychotherapy. The mental health parity measure tagged onto the 2008 bank bailout bill, which required insurers that provide mental health coverage to make that coverage equivalent to their coverage for other health conditions, was a step in the right direction, but in the effort to win over opposition from the insurance industry and business groups, it didn't go far enough. There has to be a legislative mandate, once again, so that insurers are required to provide mental health services. Health reform must make that coverage available to everyone.

To make that coverage even conceivable, and financially feasible, to guard against vast sums of money—not to mention patients' hopes and time—being wasted on questionable treatments, there also needs to be information, for insurers and for the public, on what treatments actually work.

Which means that—for economic as well as medical reasons—we have to have reliable research. We need answers regarding best practices, and we need to trust that those answers come to us from researchers and clinicians whom we can trust to have formed their opinions *independently of the drug companies.*

That's a tall order, given the insidious web of interests and alliances that currently exists between drugmakers and psychiatrists at all levels of the profession and even at the Food and Drug Administration. But it's absolutely necessary in order to establish the level of trust that parents need in order to feel comfortable in getting help for their kids and to break through one level of stigma that psychiatrists have brought upon themselves.

As I write this, there are signs that, after the scandals of the past few years, many research institutions—like Harvard Medical School, multiply embarrassed by revelations concerning some of its top child psychiatrists—are reviewing their conflict-of-interest policies, in an effort to clean up their acts. Medical schools and academic research institutions, to greatly varying degrees, have started taking steps to reduce the influence of the drug companies or at least avoid the appearance of conflict of interest. The NYU Child Study Center no longer allows drug reps to even enter the premises. The University of Pittsburgh School of Medicine has banned drug company–funded pizza lunches. The Cleveland Clinic now posts information about its doctors' relations to drug and device makers on its website. The Mayo Clinic does not permit its doctors to give drug marketing lectures.

There are national efforts under way to change the way drug research is conducted. Studies have found that industry-sponsored research is nearly four times as likely to be favorable to a company's profits as NIH-sponsored research, because of the ways that drug companies can bias their trials. Results from these tightly controlled and sometimes highly manipulated trials, some experts say, simply aren't applicable to real-world practice. Now there's a growing call by leading researchers to move away from expensive and slow industry-controlled studies that are set up to make new drugs look as good as possible (by careful screening of trial candidates, by testing new products against placebo, but not against older drugs, for example) and move toward real-world testing on populations of patients in doctors' offices, under conditions that encompass the diversity and complexity of real life.

The model for this is children's cancer research. Back in the 1970s, childhood cancer was basically a death sentence. Then researchers decided to use every bit of data available to them and started linking together all the people and places that were doing both cancer research and treatment. Every child who was treated for cancer was essentially involved in a clinical trial. Because of the wealth of evidence that was accumulated in this way over the past three decades, there is now a 90 percent cure rate for childhood cancer. Recently, the Child and Adolescent Psychiatry Trials Network, a collaboration between Duke University and the American Academy of Child and Adolescent Psychiatry, began linking hundreds of practicing child psychiatrists in just this way, planning, over a four-year period, to generate data on thousands of patients and their mental health care.

There's increasing scrutiny now within psychiatry not just of claims of drug performance garnered by industry-controlled research and of the too-cozy relationship generally that has for years existed between industry and psychiatrists, Gordon Harper, a professor of psychiatry at Harvard Medical School and medical director of Child & Adolescent Services for the Massachusetts Department of Mental Health, told me; there's now a more tempered embrace within the field of using psychotropic medication generally. There has come to be a much greater concern for the ways medications affect children's developing brains. There are more and more calls for therapeutic approaches that supplement, or even replace, medication.

"It's a paradigm shift," he said.

In many ways, it appears we've entered a period of correction.

Congress has begun considering legislation to pay health professionals to visit doctors and provide them with unbiased information on medications, in order to counteract the influence of traveling drug company sales reps. Some legislators are trying to find ways to regulate direct-to-consumer television ads for prescription medications. Senators Chuck Grassley and Herb Kohl's Physician Payments Sunshine Act of 2009 is making its way through Congress, and will require drug and device makers to publicly disclose "anything of value" that they pay or give to doctors in a national registry or else face steep fines of up to $1 million a year.

In anticipation of the bill's passage, a number of manufacturers have begun taking steps to publicly report fees and gifts to physicians, as well as educational grants and political donations. The Pharmaceutical Research and Manufacturers of America (PhRMA), in early 2009, banned gifts of pens, coffee cups, T-shirts, and other branded gifts to doctors. Much more meaningfully, the state of Massachusetts, in March 2009, banned gifts from drug and device makers to physicians, limiting when companies can pay for doctors' meals and requiring them to publicly disclose payments of over $50 to doctors for consulting and speaking on behalf of the company. The American Psychiatric Association is requiring contributors to the upcoming *DSM-V* to abide by limits on the outside compensation they can receive from drug and device makers.

As of this writing, it looks likely that the Physician Payments Sunshine Act will win passage. But as a report sponsored by the American Board of Internal Medicine Foundation and the Institute on Medicine as a Profession in 2006 pointed out, disclosure may not be enough. There are no guarantees that disclosures will be accurate. Public disclosure registries may not give patients all the information they need to discern whether or not a doctor's relationship with a drug company really amounts to a problematic conflict of interest. And, the authors of the report noted, if disclosure becomes an end in itself, it could leave many more probing questions unanswered. "Disclosure may be used to 'sanitize' a problematic situation, suggesting that no ill effects will follow from the disclosed relationship," they wrote. "Rather than eliminate the conflict, it is easier to disclose it and then proceed as though it did not exist."

The only way to truly protect consumers, they said, was to prohibit the actual practices that create conflicts of interest.

This means an iron wall between the marketing practices of drug companies and the medical practices of doctors. No more exciting trips, fancy restaurant meals, sporting event tickets. Stringent regulations on how drug samples are used and distributed. Continuing medical education that isn't funded by industry. No more medical journal articles ghostwritten by PR firms. Limitations on speaking and consulting.

We need more public funding of drug trials. And we need ethical rules to govern how industry and the research community can collaborate so that academic research centers can be trusted to produce reliable and unbiased studies.

"We ought to have as an absolute rule that once a grant is given the company should have no control over the design of the trial, the writing of the paper, the publication of the paper. It used to be that way. You'd still have the sponsorship of research. It's just that the terms of the sponsorship would be different. No more speakers bureaus, consulting arrangements. It's the marketing that would be cut off, not the research," Marcia Angell told me.

And there need to be binding rules for individual physicians and research institutions regarding financial disclosures, with penalties for noncompliance. Because, experience has shown, voluntary guidelines just don't work.

"Doctors need to reclaim certain aspects of their profession," Eric Campbell, associate professor of medicine at the Institute for Health Policy at Massachusetts General Hospital and Harvard Medical School, said. "The drug companies play an important role. But what medicine needs to do is take back control of the research, control of the education about that research. And industry needs to do truth in advertising."

The pharmaceutical industry's direct-to-consumer advertising simply ought to stop. Or, at the very least, it should be much more tightly regulated by the federal government. It used to be. Prior to 1997, the pharmaceutical industry didn't advertise much on TV, because the FDA required broadcast advertisements to include full information about drug side effects. This changed when the Food and Drug Administration Modernization Act (which also loosened regulations on off-label drug promotion) altered the rules for broadcast ads so that advertisers had only to mention major side effects and refer viewers to their doctors or to a toll-free number.

In the wake of this legislative change, spending by the pharmaceutical industry increased exponentially, nearly tripling from 1997 to 2001 alone. In this same period, pressures on physicians to prescribe specific drugs they didn't necessarily feel were medically warranted increased greatly, too, fueled by patient demand.

TV and print ads have played a large role in feeding perceptions that children's and adults' mental health conditions are trivial concerns, or merely unpleasant aspects of normal life that have been hyped up into disorders. The symptoms of mental disorders broadcast in drug ads really do sound indistinguishable from everyday problems. ("Is she depressed, Mommy?" my then eight-year-old daughter Emilie asked me one day when I told her that a friend of mine was "having a hard time," a few months after I'd broken down and signed up for cable TV, introducing her to the world of commercials. "Because depression," she piped up, "is a treatable disease.")

Who wouldn't like to have children who sit right down and do their homework with a smile, as the ads for ADHD drugs promise to deliver? Who doesn't sometimes feel overwhelmed and weary, who doesn't sometimes fantasize about finding just the right sort of instant pick-me-up that antidepressants parade as on TV? While reputable psychiatrists make distinctions in their office practice between levels of suffering or nonoptimal functioning that are "normal" and those that are severe enough to warrant treatment, advertisements don't. Yet, right now, it's the ads that are teaching many Americans about psychiatric disorders and their treatment, which means it's the drug companies that are setting the terms of the public debate.

No wonder there's so much outcry about inadequate boundaries being drawn between real and false problems. Advertising has created the appearance of reality.

If there's a "paradigm shift" happening in academia, it isn't trickling out very well into the mainstream. Too many children are still receiving substandard care. And too many people are clinging to attitudes that basically guarantee that that care will never improve.

There is still a poisonous degree of stigma surrounding the whole issue of children with mental health issues, whether it's the prejudice that seeps into the way so many people speak about these kids or the horrifically punitive way many schools engaged in "mainstreaming" now treat them, physically restraining them, locking them into seclusion rooms, sometimes seriously, even fatally, injuring them in the process.

There's still a painful degree of ignorance about what mental illness is, what it means. There is a focus on behavior—bad behavior—which is dealt with moralistically, rather than therapeutically. There is an obsession with bad parenting, which is pontificated about endlessly.

Things could be very different. If we as a society were truly interested in improving the lot of the kids we fear are being "drugged" to survive in our unnatural age, we could listen to what science now teaches about what's truly deleterious for children in our time and use that knowledge to create the best environments possible for them.

Does that mean we have the power to create or cure mental illness simply by how we organize our society and go about our lives? No. But we can make things better or worse for kids with (or without) mental health issues.

There are serious discussions to be had on childhood in our society today. There is serious work that could be done to make it less toxic and pathological. But that discussion, that challenge, is not the same as the issue of what to do to help children with mental disorders.

This distinction must be made, and it must be strengthened. And then the conversation can go forward.

A few months after finishing the bulk of this book, I watched a highly disturbing documentary on HBO called *Boy Interrupted.* It told the story of Evan Perry, a boy who was diagnosed with bipolar disorder in fifth grade and committed suicide at age fifteen, a few months after he stopped taking lithium.

Evan's was a horrible story, excruciating to watch, rendered all the more intimate by the fact that his mother, a professional filmmaker, was the documentary's director. She had photographed and videotaped him all his life—in part, she said, to concretely track the course of his illness, which had been so hard to explain to people outside of the family.

There were many devastating details to Evan's story: His father had, thirty years earlier, lost a brother to suicide. His mother, on the last night of his life, had fought with him bitterly over homework. He had been doing so well before stopping his medication that his psychiatrist had come to wonder whether he was bipolar at all.

All of this was heart-wrenching to see. Yet there was one other detail—a trivial detail—that seared me to the quick, making me feel, in the blink of an eye, like a mere spectator-observer no longer. It was the insignia on one of Evan's T-shirts.

It was the same insignia that I had on a very old camp T-shirt, saved as a souvenir of the cherished months I'd spent, decades before, living in tents on a lake. My older daughter now attended that same sleepaway camp; in fact, she'd returned home only the previous week.

Glimpsing this was like being hit with a bolt of lightning. The sight of that shirt stripped away all the layers of distance that separated me from the Perrys. I felt like there had been a death in my own family.

When the feeling passed and I looked back on it (guiltily at first, with annoyance—was it mere self-indulgence, I wondered, to make such a drama of a story not my own?) I realized that something important had happened in the moment of spotting that T-shirt. The otherness in which I—like most people—normally cloak the families of children with serious mental health issues had dissolved. And without it, I was terribly vulnerable.

That otherness is like a protective charm. It creates a shield, making it impossible for awful things, like a child's suicide, to ever happen to someone like me. We all shield ourselves like this from the full painful reality of children's mental illness all the time. We do it, in large measure, by clinging to false, simplistic, reassuring beliefs: that a child's severe separation anxiety is caused by the fact that his mother works, for example. Or that another child's ADHD is the result of too much television-watching and chocolate milk. Or that a teen's suicide is the result of insidious family dramas far worse than any that could ever roil our home. With these judgments—these magical self-incantations—we cast little fate-repelling spells: We are better parents, our children are better cared for, all will be fine.

Many of our prejudices regarding children with mental health issues, I've now come to think, may spring from this source: a deep, unavowed desire to convince ourselves that we and our children live on a separate shore from those with mental illness—and that the gulf between us and "them" will never be bridged. This desire for self-protection is understandable. No one wants to be threatened with the possibility of a life-shaking tragedy like the one that befell the Perrys. But turning our backs on the realities faced by such parents, in fact, protects no one. It just leaves everyone more vulnerable.

We are very fortunate to live in an age when documentaries like *Boy Interrupted* exist and when advocates push hard to keep the issue of children's mental illness at the forefront of our consciousness, challenging us, making us uncomfortable, making us, sometimes, bear some of the pain that families of mentally ill children formerly suffered only in private, and often in secret.

The debates over children's mental health in our time are sometimes angry, and often ugly. But there is one unequivocal bright spot in this changing, confusing landscape, where the discussion of kids' "issues" seems never to end. And it is this: However haltingly, however imperfectly, we have started to take steps that will greatly reduce the chances that if, forty years from now, a man like Richard is rediscovered at a high school reunion and asked if he thought he'd had ADHD as a child, he'll respond, "Yes—and no one ever gave a damn."

Acknowledgments

I began this book with a dedication to my husband and children, and it is to them, once again, that I must first return to express my profound and humble gratitude. The odyssey of writing this book was one that captured and burdened them as well as me, and they cheered me on selflessly and unconditionally. I must also, as always, thank my mother, Zelda Warner, whose stores of love and help are endless.

I am supremely grateful, too, to my agent, Jennifer Rudolph Walsh, whose belief in me has been greatly sustaining when my own has flagged, and who has been a tireless advocate on my behalf.

Jake Morrissey was saintlike in his patience and fortitude and, while waiting those long years for this book, became a good friend. I am very grateful as well to Geoff Kloske for his warm support and good humor over these many years, and will always be indebted to Cindy Spiegel and Susan Lehman for having brought me to Riverhead and having acquired this book in the first place. And thank you to Claire Winecoff for her careful reading and to Sarah Bowlin for making it all come together.

I am extremely grateful, too, to my editors at *The New York Times* for repeatedly giving me time off to focus on this book, encouraging me to explore its themes in my columns, and cheering my way toward the finish line.

The number of people whose voices and perspectives were essential to the creation of this book exceeds one hundred, and most can't be named here, as they shared their stories on the condition of anonymity. My most heartfelt thanks go to them.

I am extremely thankful as well for the work of the *New York Times* reporters Benedict Carey and Gardiner Harris, upon whose reporting I relied greatly while writing about the pharmaceutical industry in this book. Many doctors, researchers, and other experts were extremely generous with their time. I will try to name here those who helped, and I apologize in advance if there are any I have missed.

I want to say thank you to: Marcia Angell, Russell Barkley, Chris Bellonci, Ronald T. Brown, Eric Campbell, Larry Diller, William J. Doherty, Greg Duncan, William Frankenberger, Rosalie Greenberg, Roy Richard Grinker, Gerald N. Grob, Ned Hallowell, Gordon Peacock Harper, Thomas Insel, Jerome Kagan, Dan Kindlon, Perri Klass, Harold Koplewicz, Dana Kornfeld, Peter Kramer, Ellen Leibenluft, Madeline Levine, Mel Levine, Mindy Lewis, Suniya Luthar, Peter Jensen, Aimee Liu, Joseph Mahoney, Michael Males, John March, Steven Mintz, Wendy Mogel, Kathy Moore, Mark Olfson, Demitri Papolos, William Pelham, Daniel Pine, Kristin Kroeger Ptakowski, Judy Rapoport, John Ratey, Elizabeth Roberts, Alvin Rosenfeld, Keith Saylor, David Shaffer, Philip Shaw, William Stixrud, Don Vereen, Ben Vitiello, and Peter Whybrow.

I also owe a special debt of gratitude to Margaret O'Connell, for her generous help with final-stage research.

Notes

Preface

Page

1 In the news: Shankar Vedantam, "Debate Over Drugs for ADHD Reignites," *The Washington Post*, March 27, 2009, p. A1.

1 Three Harvard child psychiatrists: Gardiner Harris, "Three Researchers at Harvard Are Named in Subpoena," *The New York Times*, March 28, 2009, p. A9.

2 Rush Limbaugh: Cited in Michael Fumento, "Trick Question: A Liberal Hoax Turns Out to Be True," *The New Republic*, February 2, 2003.

Chapter 1: UNTITLED on Affluent Parents and Neurotic Kids

11 "Healthy but unruly children": Carol Marbin Miller, "Use of Drugs to Control Kids Worries Specialists," *The Miami Herald*, July 2, 2001, p. A1.

11 "Pills or Patience": Dorsey Griffith, "Pills or Patience: More Children Are Being Given Drugs for Behavioral and Emotional Problems," *The Sacramento Bee*, June 23, 2002, p. A1.

11 "The Antidepressant Dilemma": Jonathan Mahler, "The Antidepressant Dilemma," *The New York Times Magazine*, November 21, 2004, p. 59.

11 Prescription rates for antidepressants . . . more than tripled: Ibid., p. 59.

11 Stimulant use had quadrupled: So that, by 1996, 2.4 percent of children were taking them. Mark Olfson, Steven C. Marcus, Myrna M. Weissman, Peter S. Jensen, "National Trends in the Use of Psychotropic Medications by Children," *Journal of the American Academy of Child & Adolescent Psychiatry*, Vol. 41 (5), May 2002.

11 Antidepressant use had also tripled: From 0.3 percent of kids in 1987 to 1 percent in 1996. Mark Olfson, Steven C. Marcus, Myrna M. Weissman, and Peter S. Jensen, "National Trends in the Use of Psychotropic Medications by Children," *Journal of the American Academy of Child & Adolescent Psychiatry*, Vol. 41 (5), May 2002.

11 The use of anticonvulsant medications . . . had nearly doubled: From .35 to .69 percent. Enid M. Hunkeler et al., "Trends in Use of Antidepressants, Lithium, and Anticonvulsants in Kaiser Permanente–Insured Youths, 1994–2003," *Journal of Child and Adolescent Psychopharmacology*, Volume 15 (1), 2005, pp. 26–37.

11 Children's use of atypical antipsychotics . . . had increased fivefold: Carmen Moreno et al., "National Trends in the Outpatient Diagnosis and Treatment of Bipolar Disorder in Youth," *Archives of General Psychiatry*, Vol. 64 (9), September 2007, pp. 1032–39.

11 "Culture of intervention": Ralph Gardner, Jr., "Tot Therapy," *New York*, April 19, 2004, p. 34.

11 "Therapyland": Cathy Trost, "Enter the Therapy Zone," *The Washington Post*, November 30, 2004, p. HE01.

12 Ritalin use . . . we repeatedly read, had gone up 600 percent: See, for example, Robert Rinearson, "Our Children Suffer When We Try to Medicate Their Troubles Away," *Fort Wayne News Sentinel*, April 3, 2006. Debunking and taking apart the media frenzy on this: Daniel J. Safer, Julie M. Zito, and Eric M. Fine, "Increased Methylphenidate Usage for Attention Deficit Disorder in the 1990s," *Pediatrics*, Vol. 98 (6), December 1996, pp. 1084–88.

13 20 percent of white fifth-grade boys were on stimulant drugs: Griffith, "Pills or Patience," p. A1.

13 "Age of Ritalin": Nancy Gibbs, "The Age of Ritalin," *Time*, November 30, 1998, p. 86.

13 Harris . . . had stopped taking the drug: Jeremy Manier, "Doctors: Prozac, Violence Rarely Linked; Experts Doubtful That Halting Medication Led Directly to

Shooting at NIU," *Chicago Tribune*, February 19, 2008. Also see: Nancy Gibbs and Timothy Roche, "The Columbine Tapes," *Time*, December 20, 1999.

13 SmithKline Beecham . . . had withheld clinical findings: Wayne Kondro and Barbara Sibbald, "Drug Company Experts Advised Staff to Withhold Data About SSRI Use in Children," *Canadian Medical Association Journal*, Vol. 170 (5), March 2, 2004, p. 783.

14 Dangerous antipsychotics instead: In the wake of the black box warning on antidepressants, some physicians began switching children from those drugs to antipsychotic drugs, none of which were approved for children. Thomas Insel, director of the National Institute of Mental Health, worried, "Have we gone from one set of medications of known benefit and of questionable risks to a group of medications with unknown benefits and well-known risks?" Quoted in Shankar Vedantam, "Psychiatric Drugs' Use Drops for Children," *The Washington Post*, October 8, 2005, p. A1.

14 Preschoolers . . . were now being given psychotropic drugs: Julie Magno Zito et al., "Trends in the Prescribing of Psychotropic Medications to Preschoolers," *JAMA*, Vol. 283, 2000, pp. 1025–30. Cited in http://www.pbs.org/wgbh/pages/frontline/shows/medicating/drugs/dontknow.html.

14 Breggin testimony to Congress: http://www.breggin.com/congress.html.

14 Parents alleging that schools were threatening to kick children out: "First-of-its-Kind Law Bars Schools from Recommending Meds," *Mental Health Weekly*, August 6, 2001, p. 3.

15 For conservatives fearful of government intrusion, see, for example: Phyllis Schlafly, "No Child Left Unmedicated," *The Phyllis Schlafly Report*, Vol. 38 (8), March 2005.

15 On attempt to "feminize" boys: Suzanne Fields, "Disappearing Acts; How Males Became the 'Second Sex,'" *The Washington Times*, May 29, 2003.

15 The "sorcery" of psychiatrists: Alexander Cockburn, "But the Pills Your Mother Gives You . . ." *Counterpunch*, April 2–3, 2005.

15 The "medicopharmaceutical industrial complex": Richard DeGrandpre, *The Cult of Pharmacology: How America Became the World's Most Troubled Drug Culture* (Durham: Duke University Press, 2006), p. 170.

15 "Doped up": Angelica Rosas, "Vince Vaughn Just Says No to Ritalin with 'Thumbsucker,'" mtv.com, July 23, 2004.

16 "It may be a clue": Barbara Ehrenreich, "What's the Matter with Kids Today?" *The New York Times Book Review*, May 9, 2004, p. 9.

17 "Arguably inhuman rhythms": Mary Eberstadt, *Home-Alone America: The Hidden Toll of Day Care, Behavioral Drugs, and Other Parent Substitutes* (New York: Sentinel, 2004), p. 78.

21 "This destructive force": Address by Alvin Rosenfeld, "The Over-Scheduled Family," St. Luke's School, November 15, 2006. http://www.hyper-parenting.com/talkstluke.htm.

23 "Dr. Breggin's observations are totally without credibility": Order and Decision from Proceedings held before the Honorable James W. Rice, Reserved Circuit Court Judge Presiding, Case No. 93-FA-939-763, *Jacqueline D. Schellinger v. Neal C. Schellinger*, July 2, 1997, pp. 70–71.

23 Utterly inarticulate: judging by her appearance on "A Parent's Right to Choose: Guests Discuss the Issue of Children Being Medicated to Treat Behavioral Problems," *The Montel Williams Show*, April 15, 2003.

24 SSRIs created modern depression: David Healy, *Let Them Eat Prozac: The Unhealthy Relationship Between the Pharmaceutical Industry and Depression* (New York: New York University Press 2004), p. 4 ff.

24 "Liberating patients": David Healy, *The Creation of Psychopharmacology* (Cambridge: Harvard University Press, 2002), p. 175.

24 "Mental illness is the revolt": Cited in ibid., p. 151.

26 "Zealot-researchers have seized the history of psychiatry": Edward Shorter, *A History of Psychiatry: From the Era of the Asylum to the Age of Prozac* (New York: John Wiley & Sons, 1997), p. viii. Shorter, Healy, and other writers now maintain that Foucault simply got a lot of his facts wrong. For an additional example, see Andrew Scull, "The Fictions of Foucault's Scholarship," *Times Literary Supplement*, March 21, 2007.

26 Deinstitutionalization as humanitarian disaster: Shorter, p. 280.

Chapter 2: Seeing Is Believing

31 "If I didn't believe": Author interview.

32 At least 25 percent of American adults suffer to some degree from a mental disorder: According to Ronald C. Kessler et al., "Lifetime Prevalence and Age-of-Onset Distributions of *DSM-IV* Disorders in the National Comorbidity Survey Replication," *Archives of General Psychiatry*, Vol. 62, June 2005, pp. 593–602, almost half of all adults surveyed were said to suffer from mental health issues se-

vere enough to qualify as diagnosable disorders at some point in their lives. Nearly 29 percent of adults would at some point suffer from anxiety disorders, almost 21 percent from mood disorders, nearly 25 percent from impulse control disorders, nearly 15 percent from substance use disorders, and nearly 17 percent from major depressive disorder. Kessler et al. argue that their figures are conservative, as the study excluded the homeless and people in institutions, and people tend to underreport embarrassing things like mental illness to pollsters.

32 About half of those people are affected enough to need treatment: And suffer at least moderate impairments in their work and in their lives. Ronald C. Kessler, Wai Tat Chiu, Olga Demler, and Ellen E. Walters, "Prevalence, Severity, and Comorbidity of 12-Month *DSM-IV* Disorders in the National Comorbidity Survey Replication," *Archives of General Psychiatry,* Vol. 62, June 2005, pp. 617–627.

32 Six percent are so impaired that they attempt suicide or live at "substantial limitations": Ibid., pp. 617–627. Close to 7 percent more are subject to "moderate" impairments in work and life that can rise to the level of thinking about or planning for suicide.

32 33 million people were prescribed at least one psychiatric drug: Charles Barber, *Comfortably Numb* (New York: Vintage, 2008), p. 8.

33 More than half . . . began to have symptoms as children: The National Comorbidity Survey in 2005 found that more than half of the adults with serious psychiatric illnesses had begun to suffer from the symptoms of their disorders by the time they were fourteen. The median age of onset for anxiety and "impulse control disorders" was age eleven. (Ronald C. Kessler et al., "Lifetime Prevalence and Age-of-Onset Distributions of *DSM-IV* Disorders in the National Comorbidity Survey Replication," *Archives of General Psychiatry,* Vol. 62, June 2005, pp. 593–602.)

Other recent research suggests that this 50 percent rate of childhood onset for adult mental disorders may actually be understated. According to the National Institute of Mental Health's Daniel Pine, a specialist in mood and anxiety disorders, about two-thirds of adults who suffer from mental illness have at least some antecedents in childhood. "If you look at affected adults between the ages of twenty and forty who have depression, you would find about 60 percent of them, if you had seen them as kids, would have had a clearly identifiable mental health problem," he told me in an interview. About half of kids with mental health issues somehow outgrow them prior to adulthood, he said. But the ones with more severe problems generally don't. "Problems are very common in kids;

they're usually transient, but the group of kids with persistent problems will grow up to be a lot of the adults with problems."

36 The number of children receiving diagnoses of mental disorders has tripled: Benedict Carey, "Your Child's Disorder May Be Yours, Too," *The New York Times*, December 9, 2007.

36 "If children cough after exercising": H. Gilbert Welch, Lisa Schwartz, and Steven Woloshin, "What's Making Us Sick Is an Epidemic of Diagnoses," *The New York Times*, January 2, 2007.

36 Higher than could be normally expected outbreaks: An "epidemic," according to the Centers for Disease Control and Prevention, is "the occurrence of more cases of disease than expected in a given area or among a specific group of people over a particular period of time."

36 "Something's rotten": Lidia Wasowicz, "Ped Med: Young Minds Under Attack," United Press International, January 9, 2006.

36 A major national survey: Ronald C. Kessler et al., "Lifetime Prevalence and Age-of-Onset Distributions of *DSM-IV* Disorders in the National Comorbidity Survey Replication," *Archives of General Psychiatry*, Vol. 62, June 2005, pp. 593–602.

37 "Fidgety Phil": Cited in "Attention Deficit Hyperactivity Disorder: From Genes to Patients," *The New England Journal of Medicine*, Vol. 354 (2), May 18, 2006, p. 2198.

37 Emil Kraepelin observations: Jon McClellan and John Werry, "Practice Parameters for the Assessment and Treatment of Children and Adolescents with Bipolar Disorder," *Journal of the American Academy of Child & Adolescent Psychiatry*, Vol. 36, (1), 1997, pp. 138–57.

37 Asylum psychiatrists: Ibid.

38 The Freudians believed: Demitri and Janice Papolos, *The Bipolar Child* (New York: Broadway Books, 2002), p. 26.

38 They similarly believed: Ibid., pp. 26–27.

38 "Minimal brain dysfunction": Kevin T. Kalikow, *Your Child in the Balance: An Insider's Guide for Parents to the Psychiatric Medication Dilemma* (New York: Perseus, 2006), p. 61.

38 Children's mental health diagnoses in Freudian era: American Psychiatric Association, *Diagnostic and Statistical Manual: Mental Disorders*, 1952, p. 40 ff.

38 Behavior Disorders of Childhood and Adolescence: American Psychiatric Association, *Diagnostic and Statistical Manual of Mental Disorders, Second Edition*, 1968, p. 49 ff.

39 "Autistic atypical and withdrawn behavior": *DSM-II*, p. 35.

40 "You are making the problem worse": Anne Ford, *Laughing Allegra* (New York: Newmarket Press, 2003), p. 41.

40 "Acute schizophrenic reaction": Mindy Lewis, *Life Inside* (New York: Atria, 2002), pp. 4–18.

41 Psychologist Wendy Mogel: Author interview, September 13, 2006.

41 On the psychologization of learning disabilities: One prominent child psychopathology textbook author, as late as 1988, lamented her profession's shift in focus from "psychological" to "organic" causes of learning difficulties. "In recent years, the term 'underachiever' has been replaced by 'learning disability,'" she wrote. "In the past ten years or so, learning disabilities have been studied as psychoneurological or cognitive dysfunctions, ignoring more general personality issues. This is probably a mistake." Jane W. Kessler, *Psychopathology of Childhood,* Second Edition (Englewood Cliffs, NJ: Prentice Hall, 1988), pp. 385–386 and p. 372.

41 When Diller proposed treating the boy with behavioral techniques: Lawrence H. Diller, *Should I Medicate My Child?* (New York: Basic Books, 2002), p. 18.

42 The drugs . . . made their bodies rigid: Interview with Ben Vitiello, chief of the Child and Adolescent Treatment and Preventive Intervention Research Branch at the National Institute of Mental Health, November 21, 2008.

42 David Shaffer: Author interview. May 28, 2008.

43 A rebellion against Freudianism: Notably among the "neo-Kraepelians," largely centered in the psychiatry department at Washington University in Saint Louis, who were interested in brain chemistry and neurobiology. They were eager to produce a classification system for mental disorders based on checklists of symptoms rather than on the underlying conflicts that the Freudians believed the symptoms expressed. See Edward Shorter, *A History of Psychiatry: From the Era of the Asylum to the Age of Prozac* (New York: John Wiley & Sons, 1997), p. 300.

43 Many doctors now believed that psychoanalysis simply didn't work for patients other than mildly affected neurotics: In the early 1950s, Hans Eysenck, director of the psychological department of Maudsley Hospital in London, had compared outcome studies of patients treated with psychoanalysis and other therapies. Only 44 percent of those treated with psychoanalysis improved by the end of therapy, he found. Simply letting time pass, on the other hand, was shown to cure fully two-thirds of "neurotic" patients—as nonpsychotics were called—within two years, notes Edward Shorter, p. 312.

43 The discovery of chlorpromazine: Through clinical trials. See Healy, *The Creation of Psychopharmacology,* p. 100.

43 Resistance from the psychoanalytic establishment: Shorter, p. 257 ff.

45 Harold Koplewicz: Author interview. May 2, 2008.

45 Child and teen depression recognized as such in the mid-1970s: Papolos, p. 26 ff.

45 First generation of antidepressants . . . weren't effective in children: Mark Olfson, Steven C. Marcus, Myrna M. Weissman, Peter S. Jensen, "National Trends in the Use of Psychotropic Medications by Children," *Journal of the American Academy of Child and Adolescent Psychiatry*, Vol. 41 (5), May 2002.

45 Benzedrine used since 1930s: Child and teen depression recognized as such in mid 1970s: Cited in Carla Garnett, "Attention Deficit, Hyperactivity Explored in Depth at STEP Forum," NIH Record, Vol. LVIII, (4), February 24, 2006.

46 "Physicians prefer to diagnose conditions they can treat": Shorter, p. 291.

47 The average pediatric stay on a psych ward: Paul Raeburn, *Acquainted with the Night: A Parent's Quest to Understand Depression and Bipolar Disorder in His Children* (New York: Broadway Books, 2005), p. 139.

47 "Almost a million children with disabilities": Steven Mintz, *Huck's Raft: A History of American Childhood* (Cambridge: Belknap Press, 2004), p. 324.

47 "Checklist for Camp": Jane Gross, "Checklist for Camp: Bug Spray. Sunscreen. Pills," *The New York Times*, July 16, 2006.

47 "Young Minds Under Attack": Lidia Wasowicz, "Ped Med: Young Minds Under Attack," United Press International, January 9, 2006.

Chapter 3: An Epidemic of Supposition

49 "A public health crisis"/ "flavor of the month": "A Mind of Their Own," *American RadioWorks*, American Public Media, April 19, 2005.

49 One in 2,000 to 5,000: First range is from Paul T. Shattuck and Maureen Durkin, "A Spectrum of Disputes," *The New York Times*, June 11, 2007, p. A19. Second range is from http://www.nimh.nih.gov/health/publications/autism/introduction.shtm.

50 Fewer than three in 10,000: Roy Richard Grinker, *Unstrange Minds: Remapping the World of Autism* (Cambridge: Basic Books, 2007), p. 8.

50 Former diagnoses for children who would today be called autistic: Ibid., p. 16.

50 One third more children categorized with autism spectrum disorders: Bryna Siegel, *Helping Children with Autism Learn: Treatment Approaches for Parents and Professionals* (New York: Oxford University Press, 2003), p. 14.

50 A 3,500 percent increase: Paul T. Shattuck and Maureen Durkin, "A Spectrum of Disputes," *The New York Times*, June 11, 2007, p. A19.

52 Two to fifteen percent of kids: Estimates of the prevalence of depression in children range from a conservative figure of 2 percent cited repeatedly by psychiatric researchers, to the most liberal figure, from the Department of Health and Human Services, which allows that 10 to 15 percent of children and adolescents show "*some* symptoms of depression" at any given point in time. Two percent: Melissa A. Brotman et al., "Prevalence, Clinical Correlates, and Longitudinal Course of Severe Mood Dysregulation in Children," *Biological Psychiatry*, Vol. 60, 2006, pp. 991–997. Ten to fifteen percent: http://mentalhealth.samhsa.gov/publications/allpubs/CA-0011/default.asp#1.

52 Up to one percent: Carey Goldberg, "Bipolar Labels for Children Stir Concern," *The Boston Globe*, February 15, 2007.

52 1.5 to 2 percent of school-aged children were taking stimulants: "Either Ritalin or Dexedrine." Jane W. Kessler, *Psychopathology of Childhood*, Second Edition (Englewood Cliffs, NJ: Prentice Hall, 1988), p. 342.

52 ADHD is believed to be present in about 8 percent of kids: Data analyzed by the Centers for Disease Control and Prevention from its 2003 National Survey of Children's Health, a phone survey of the parents or guardians of 102,353 children, found 7.8 percent of children aged four to seventeen having been diagnosed with ADHD (http://www.cdc.gov/ncbddd/ADHD/). More recently, a July 2008 report from the CDC and the National Center for Health Statistics, put the prevalence of ADHD at 8.4 percent of children aged six to seventeen. That report cited other major studies putting ADHD prevalence at 7.8 percent and 8.2 percent or as high as 8.7 percent in another study, which determined how many children met *DSM-IV* criteria for ADHD according to parent reports of their behavior. The latter was Froelich et al., "Prevalence, recognition, and treatment of attention-deficit/hyperactivity disorder in a national sample of U.S. children," *Archives of Pediatric and Adolescent Psychiatry*, Vol. 161, 2007, pp. 857–64. Cited in Patricia N. Pastor and Cynthia A. Reuben, "Diagnosed Attention Deficit Hyperactivity Disorder and Learning Disability: United States, 2004–2006," National Center for Health Statistics, Vital and Health Statistics, Series 10, No. 237, July 2008.

52 Epidemiologists say: James M. Perrin, Sheila R. Bloom, Steven L. Gortmaker, "Increasing Childhood Chronic Conditions in the United States," *JAMA*, Vol. 297 (24), June 27, 2007, pp. 1–4.

52 The arguments about changed diagnosing patterns and the effect of IDEA are also present in: Mark Olfson, Marc J. Gameroff, Steven C. Marcus, and Peter S. Jensen, "National Trends in the Treatment of Attention Deficit Hyperactivity Disorder," *American Journal of Psychiatry*, Vol. 160 (6), June 2003, pp. 1071–77.

53 "cohort" studies: See Demitri and Janice Papolos, *The Bipolar Child* (New York: Broadway Books, 2002), p. 25. One study showed that people born around 1910 had only a 1.3 percent chance of having a major depressive episode, whereas those born after 1960 had a 5.3 percent chance, and there was an approximately tenfold increase in risk for depression in each successive generational cohort. Another study of families with depression showed higher rates of severe clinical depression in younger relatives than older ones. Both studies are also cited in Ed Diener and Martin E. P. Seligman, "Beyond Money: Toward an Economy of Well-Being," *Psychological Science in the Public Interest,* Vol. 5 (1), 2004, pp. 1–31.

53 Jean Twenge . . . made this argument: Not very convincingly, though, I thought. Twenge combines mention of the "cohort" studies, dire incidence statistics on teen and college student depression, her doctoral research on children's anxiety, and observations of her closest friends to argue that kids' anxiety is now off the charts. "I know this trend toward depression and anxiety firsthand. Among my ten closest friends," she wrote, "seven have been in therapy, at least once, two suffer from panic attacks, one is manic-depressive, and another recently had a nervous breakdown. They are college-educated, successful, and usually well-adjusted people. . . ."

Jean Twenge, *Generation Me: Why Today's Young Americans Are More Confident, Assertive, Entitled–and More Miserable Than Ever Before* (New York: Free Press, 2006), p. 107 ff.

54 Bipolar disorder is increasing and coming on much earlier in children: Papolos, p. 164.

55 "Assortative mating" and autism: Simon Baron-Cohen, "The Male Condition," *The New York Times*, August 8, 2005, p. A15.

55 "Very intense systemizing": http://www.edge.org/3rd_culture/baron-cohen05/baron-cohen05_index.html.

55 "Some evolutionary psychologists": Author interviews for Judith Warner, "Glass Sippers? Old Hat," *The New York Times*, March 10, 2007, p. A13. And for "hybrid vigor" discussion see Aimee Liu, *Gaining: The Truth About Life After Eating Disorders* (New York: Warner Books, 2007).

56 Well-off teens are outpacing their middle-class peers . . . 30 to 40 percent of affluent twelve- to eighteen-year-olds show "troubling psychological symptoms": This and previous sentence, Madeline Levine, *The Price of Privilege: How Parental Pressure and Material Advantage Are Creating a Generation of Disconnected and Unhappy Kids* (New York: HarperCollins, 2006), p. 21.

56 As many as 22 percent of well-off adolescent girls suffer from depression; one-third show anxiety: Ibid., p. 18.

56 For an extended discussion of the manic drive in our culture, see Peter C. Whybrow, *American Mania: When More Is Not Enough* (New York: W. W. Norton & Co., 2005).

56 Hard data just doesn't exist: It was in the 1970s that the use of structured interviews to collect population sample data on childhood depression began. See E. Jane Costello, Alaattin Erkanli, and Adrian Angold, "Is There an Epidemic of Child or Adolescent Depression?" *The Journal of Child Psychology and Psychiatry*, Vol. 47 (12), 2006, pp. 1263–71. "People are always claiming a disorder they're interested in has become more prevalent," Dr. David Shaffer of Columbia told me. "But in order to demonstrate that there really has been a change over time you have to use similar methods at two times and very few studies have done that because the nomenclature was changing and methods were changing. Maybe the vocabulary has changed and the use of disorders rather than psychological influences [to describe what's going on with children] has evolved," he said. "I hope we're recognizing things better and that things like blaming background is becoming more outdated. [But] I don't know about increases."

57 "Not asking . . . not having": Gabrielle A. Carlson, "Who Are the Children with Severe Mood Dysregulation, a.k.a. 'Rages'?" *The American Journal of Psychiatry*, Vol. 164, August 2007, pp. 1140–42.

57 No real increase in depression in kids: E. Jane Costello, Alaattin Erkanli, and Adrian Angold, "Is There an Epidemic of Child or Adolescent Depression?" *The Journal of Child Psychology and Psychiatry*, Vol. 47 (12), 2006, pp. 1263–71.

58 "No clear evidence documents a secular increase in prevalence of depression": James M. Perrin, Sheila R. Bloom, and Steven L. Gortmaker, "Increasing Childhood Chronic Conditions in the United States," *JAMA*, Vol. 297 (24), June 27, 2007, pp. 1–4.

58 Teen pregnancy, school violence, crime, cigarette smoking, and substance use declining: Author interview with Harvard University psychologist Dan Kindlon, author of *Too Much of a Good Thing: Raising Children of Character in an Indulgent Age*

and *Alpha Girls: Understanding the New American Girl and How She Is Changing the World.* For decreases in teen suicide (to 2003), cigarette smoking, drinking, see "Youth Risk Behavior Surveillance–United States 2005," Morbidity and Mortality Weekly Report, Department of Health and Human Services Centers for Disease Control and Prevention, Vol. 55, June 9, 2006. Also see, for decreased drugs, alcohol, cigarette use: University of Michigan Institute for Social Research, "Monitoring the Future Survey," December 2007.

58 Teen suicide rate fell 30 percent: M. Gould, T. Greenberg, D. Velting, and D. Shaffer, "Youth Suicide Risk and Preventive Interventions: A Review of the Past 10 Years, *The Journal of the American Academy of Child & Adolescent Psychiatry*, Vol. 42, 2003, pp. 386–405. Cited in E. Jane Costello, Alaattin Erkanli, and Adrian Angold, "Is There an Epidemic of Child or Adolescent Depression?" *The Journal of Child Psychology and Psychiatry*, Vol. 47 (12), 2006, pp. 1263–71.

58 Author interview with Dr. David Shaffer, May 28, 2008. Also see R. D. Gibbons et al., "Early Evidence on the Effects of Regulators' Suicidality Warnings on SSRI Prescriptions and Suicide in Children and Adolescents," *The American Journal of Psychiatry*, Vol. 164, September 2007, pp. 1356–63. The authors note that there was a 14 percent increase in the child and adolescent suicide rates in the U.S. from 2003–2004, the period in which there was considerable public discussion of the risks of SSRIs and the FDA placed its black box warning on the drugs. This was, they write, "the first increase of this magnitude in the child and adolescent suicide rate since the CDC began systematically collecting data in 1979." The authors acknowledge that prescribing rates of SSRIs to kids in that year didn't drop anywhere nearly as sharply as the suicide rate increased, but speculate that all the public health warnings "may have left some of the most vulnerable youths untreated."

59 Teenagers today miss fewer days of school, finish high school and college more than boomers: Steven Mintz, *Huck's Raft: A History of American Childhood.* (Cambridge: Belknap Press, 2004), p. 345.

59 College freshmen who find themselves "frequently depressed" declining, etc: Mike Males, "The Mental Health Crisis That Isn't," *The Los Angeles Times*, May 27, 2007.

60 Child bipolar diagnoses increased forty-fold: Carmen Moreno et al., "National Trends in the Outpatient Diagnosis and Treatment of Bipolar Disorder in Youth," *Archives of General Psychiatry*, Vol. 64, (9), September 2007, pp. 1032–39.

60 Half a million to a million: Rosalie Greenberg, *Bipolar Kids: Helping Your Child Find Calm in the Mood Storm* (Cambridge, MA: Da Capo, 2007), p. ix. According to the Department of Health and Human services, at least 750,000 children in the United States suffer from bipolar disorder. http://mentalhealth.samhsa.gov/publications/allpubs/CA-0006/default.asp#10. *60 Minutes* reported in 2007 that nearly one million children had been diagnosed as bipolar. "What Killed Rebecca Riley?" CBS News, September 30, 2007.

60 Approximately one-fourth of pediatric patients discharged from psychiatric hospitals called bipolar: Author interview with Mark Olfson, April 21, 2008.

61 Adult diagnoses are two-thirds female; child diagnoses two-thirds male: Carmen Moreno et al., "National Trends in the Outpatient Diagnosis and Treatment of Bipolar Disorder in Youth," *Archives of General Psychiatry*, Vol. 64, (9), September 2007, pp. 1032–39.

61 "A somewhat tautological undertaking": Jennifer Harris, "Child & Adolescent Psychiatry: The Increased Diagnosis of 'Juvenile Bipolar Disorder': What Are We Treating?" *Psychiatric Services*, Vol. 56, May 2005, pp. 529–31.

61 Child irritability correlates with greater later risk of anxiety and depression: Argyris Stringaris, Patricia Cohen, Daniel S. Pine, and Ellen Leibenluft, "Adult Outcomes of Youth Irritability: A 20-Year Prospective Community-Based Study," *American Journal of Psychiatry* online, July 1, 2009.

61 Westchester County study: David L. Pogge et al., "Diagnosis of manic episodes in adolescent inpatients: structured diagnostic procedures compared to clinical chart diagnoses," *Psychiatry Research*, Vol. 101, 2001, pp. 47–54.

62 Many kids with severe mood dysregulations grow up to be severely depressed: Brotman et al., "Prevalence, Clinical Correlates, and Longitudinal Course of Severe Mood Dysregulation in Children," pp. 991–97.

62 Falsely diagnosed bipolar kids got worse on anticonvulsants: Pogge et al., "Diagnosis of manic episodes in adolescent inpatients: structured diagnostic procedures compared to clinical chart diagnoses," pp. 47–54.

63 A report from the National Institute of Mental Health: *Blueprint for Change: Research on Child and Adolescent Mental Health*, Report of the National Advisory Mental Health Council Workgroup on Child and Adolescent Mental Health Intervention Development and Deployment, Washington, D.C., The National Institute of Mental Health, Office of Communications and Public Liaison, May 2001, Preface.

Chapter 4: Aren't *They All* on Medication?

65 "Legal-drugging epidemic": Arianna Huffington, "*Distracted*: a Powerful New Play Takes on Our 'Pill for Every Ill' Culture," huffingtonpost.com, April 2, 2007.

67 Ritalin prescriptions up 600 percent: Robert Rinearson, "Our Children Suffer When We Try to Medicate Their Troubles Away," *Fort Wayne News-Sentinel*, April 3, 2006.

67 18 to 20 percent of white boys taking stimulants: Dorsey Griffith, "Pills or Patience: More Children Are Being Given Drugs for Behavioral and Emotional Problems," *The Sacramento Bee*, June 23, 2002, p. A1.

68 Antidepressant prescriptions for kids under eighteen tripled: Jonathan Mahler, "The Antidepressant Dilemma," *The New York Times Magazine*, November 21, 2004, p. 59.

68 "A more than fivefold increase": Jenny Rempel, "Don't Crush Budding Einsteins," *Fresno Bee*, November 12, 2006, p. K8.

68 Psychotropic drug use . . . nearly tripled: Shari Roan, "Young and Alone," *Los Angeles Times*, February 27, 2006.

68 The alleged 600 percent increase in Ritalin use: The 600 percent increase in Ritalin use never happened. What did happen was: there was a shortage of Ritalin in 1993 that left children in some parts of the country going months without access to their medication. Subsequently, the Drug Enforcement Agency demanded a massive ramping-up of Ritalin production, so that such shortfalls wouldn't occur again. As a result of this action, the DEA's *production quotas* were shown to increase sixfold from 1990 to mid-1995. Ritalin use went up in that period, too, largely due to the longer use of stimulants by children and adults and the expanded understanding of ADHD made official in 1994 by the *DSM-IV*, but by nowhere near 600 percent. The true increase in children's Ritalin usage in that period was 2.5-fold, according to researchers Daniel J. Safer, Julie M. Zito, and Eric M. Fine, who investigated the issue for a study published in the December 1996 issue of the journal *Pediatrics*. (Daniel J. Safer, Julie M. Zito, and Eric M. Fine, "Increased Methylphenidate Usage for Attention Deficit Disorder in the 1990s," *Pediatrics*, Vol. 98 (6), December 1996, pp. 1084–88.) For DEA information, see Safer, Zito, and Fine and also Russell Barkley, "ADHD, Ritalin and Conspiracies: Talking Back to Peter Breggin," 1998, www.quackwatch.com.

68 The "fact" that up to a fifth of fifth-grade boys: The 20 percent number was generated by Gretchen B. LeFever, a researcher in the department of pediatrics

at the East Virginia Medical School. The finding was never replicated afterward, though the state of Virginia—where the huge drug use was allegedly found—tried repeatedly to do so. (State investigators found that between 1.5 and 11.4 percent of school children in various parts of the state were taking ADHD meds.) The researcher who generated those numbers was eventually charged with scientific misconduct for the way she'd conducted another study, which found a whopping 17 percent of elementary school children diagnosed with ADHD. Though she was ultimately cleared of all charges, she ended up leaving her medical school and found a home eventually on the faculty of televangelist Pat Robertston's Regent University. I am indebted, for this account, to the reporting of Bill Sizemore of *The Virginian-Pilot*. Notably his articles, "Did Study Miss the Mark?" *The Virginian-Pilot*, January 23, 2005, and "Whatever Happened to . . . the EVMS Researcher who Studied ADHD?" *The Virginian-Pilot*, August 14, 2006. Also see: Jeanne Lenzer, "Researcher Cleared of Misconduct Charges," *British Medical Journal*, October 15, 2005. And Jeanne Lenzer, "Researcher to Be Sacked After Reporting High Rates of ADHD," *British Medical Journal*, March 26, 2005.

68 The first generation drugs: On the history of antidepressant use and the fact that studies in the 1990s showed the efficacy of Prozac: Mark Olfson, Steven C. Marcus, Myrna M. Weissman, and Peter S. Jensen, "National Trends in the Use of Psychotropic Medications by Children," *Journal of the American Academy of Child & Adolescent Psychiatry*, Vol. 41 (5), May 2002. The effectiveness of SSRIs remains a matter of great media debate, but I have found the consensus among clinicians to be that they have been a godsend for many severely depressed and anxious children and teens.

68 I've seen numbers ranging from one-half of a percent to 1.3 percent: Kevin T. Kalikow, in, *Your Child in the Balance: An Insider's Guide for Parents to the Psychiatric Medication Dilemma*, New York: Perseus, 2006, p. 182, writes that between one half and one percent of children under age eighteen were taking antidepressants in the late 1990s. 1.3% of youth under age nineteen were taking antidepressants in 1997, according to Mark Olfson and Steven C. Marcus, "National Patterns in Antidepressant Medication Treatment," *Archives of General Psychiatry*, Vol. 66 (No. 8), August 2009, pp. 848–856. According to a study of Kaiser Permanente enrollees in Northern California, .94 percent of children and teens were taking antidepressants in 1994: Enid M. Hunkeler et al., "Trends in Use of Antidepressants, Lithium, and Anticonvulsants in Kaiser Permanente–Insured Youths, 1994–2003," *Journal of Child and Adolescent Psychopharmacology*, Volume 15 (1), 2005, pp. 26–37.

69 Depending on who's counting: Up to 1 or 2 percent today: Use of antidepressants by youths under nineteen years increased from 1.3 percent in 1997 to 1.8 percent in 2002, according to Olfson and Marcus. Hunkeler et al. put antidepressant use in 2003 at 2.1 percent of children and teens in the Northern California survey. Antidepressant use in children dropped nationally after 2004.

69 Depending on who's counting: The estimated prevalence of depression in kids is either 2 percent, as some researchers hold (Melissa A. Brotman et al., "Prevalence, Clinical Correlates, and Longitudinal Course of Severe Mood Dysregulation in Children," *Biological Psychiatry*, Vol. 60, 2006, pp. 991–97), or 8 percent, as other researchers say (according to Kalikow, p. 182), or 10 to 15 percent, as the U.S. government asserts, when it defines depression in the most liberal way. (The Department of Health and Human Services says that 10 to 15 percent of children and adolescents show "*some* symptoms of depression" at any given point in time. http://mentalhealth.samhsa.gov/publications/allpubs/CA-0011/default.asp#1).

69 A "chemical sledgehammer": David Crary, "A Dilemma: Medications for Foster Kids," Associated Press, March 13, 2007. And Michelle Cole and Brent Walth, "Foster Kids, Meds Merit Exam," *The Oregonian*, November 27, 2007.

69 As many as 60 percent of foster kids . . . and less than half: Cited in Ramesh Raghavan et al., "Psychotropic Medication Use in a National Probability Sample of Children in the Child Welfare System," *Journal of Child and Adolescent Psychopharmacology*, Vol. 15 (1), 2005, pp. 97–106.

69 One in four cases in the state of Virginia: "Improving the Quality of Health Care for Mental and Substance-Use Conditions," a report of the Institute of Medicine, 2006.

70 About two-thirds of the inmates: Solomon Moore, "Mentally Ill Offenders Strain Juvenile System," *The New York Times*, August 10, 2009.

70 Five percent of kids: According to the Centers for Disease Control and Prevention, approximately 5 percent of children age four to seventeen take medication for difficulties with emotions or behavior. See Gloria Simpson et al., "Use of Mental Health Services in the Past 12 Months by Children aged 4–17 Years: United States, 2005–2006," NCHS Data Brief, No. 8, September 2008.

71 5 to 20 percent have psychiatric issues: *Mental Health: A Report of the Surgeon General*. Rockville, MD: Department of Health and Human Services, Substance Abuse and Mental Health Services Administration, Center for Mental Health Services, National Institute of Mental Health, 1999, The American Academy of Pediatrics and the NYU Child Study Center.

71 86 percent of Americans: Bernice A. Pescosolido, Brea L. Perry, Jack K. Martin, and Jane D. McLoed, "Stigmatizing Attitudes and Beliefs About Treatment and Psychiatric Medications for Children with Mental Illness" *Psychiatric Services*, Vol. 58 (5) May 2007, pp. 613–18.

72 3.3 percent of children: This is Froelich et al., "Prevalence, recognition, and treatment of attention-deficit/hyperactivity disorder in a national sample of U.S. children," *Archives of Pediatric and Adolescent Psychiatry*, Vol. 161, 2007, pp. 857–64. Cited in Patricia N. Pastor and Cynthia A. Reuben, "Diagnosed Attention Deficit Hyperactivity Disorder and Learning Disability: United States, 2004–2006," National Center for Health Statistics, Vital and Health Statistics, Series 10, No. 237, July 2008.

72 Underdiagnosis and underuse of medication: Ibid. In this study, 8.7 percent of eight- to fifteen-year-olds overall did meet the criteria for ADHD, but only 50 percent of the kids who met the *DSM-IV* criteria for ADHD had ever been formally diagnosed with the disorder. A 2007 study, published in the *Archives of Pediatrics and Adolescent Medicine*, which measured prevalence by interviewing 3,082 caregivers using the *DSM-IV* criteria for ADHD, found that, while 8.7 percent of children met the criteria, only 47.9 percent of those children had been diagnosed with the disorder. Only a third of girls who met the ADHD criteria had been diagnosed with the disorder. And only 38.8 percent of the children who met the ADHD criteria had received treatment with medication in the prior year. (Larissa Hirsch and Charles A. Pohl, "ADHD: More Prevalent Than We Thought?" psychiatrictimes.com, October 1, 2007.)

72 Only about half of kids with ADHD get any treatment: In 2003, according to the Centers for Disease Control and Prevention 56 percent of the children who had been diagnosed with ADHD were taking medication for the disorder (http://www.cdc.gov/ncbddd/ADHD/). Similarly, a 2007 study in the *Journal of Attention Disorders* found, using pharmacy claims data for a large population of Americans with private health insurance, that in 2005, 4.4 percent of children were using ADHD medications—again, about 50 percent of kids with ADHD. (Castle et al., "Trends in Medication Treatment for ADHD," *Journal of Attention Disorders*, 2007, Vol. 10, 2007, pp. 335–42.)

72 Studies routinely find: The professional consensus on ADHD treatment was summed up, in 2007, by a survey on public knowledge, beliefs, and treatment preferences concerning ADHD in the journal *Psychiatric Services:* "Research on treatment utilization suggests that only half of children with ADHD receive treat-

ment, and less than half of them receive specialty care. Fewer children receive psychostimulant medications than would be expected with estimated population prevalence rates, which supports the claim that ADHD is underdiagnosed and undertreated." (Jane D. McLeod, Danielle L. Fettes, Peter S. Jensen, Bernice A. Pescosolido, and Jack K. Martin, "Public Knowledge, Beliefs, and Treatment Preferences Concerning Attention-Deficit Hyperactivity Disorder," *Psychiatric Services*, Vol. 58, (5), May 2007, pp. 626–31.)

72 A problematic amount of geographical variation: This was the finding of a massive 2003 study conducted by the Centers for Disease Control and Prevention which surveyed the parents and guardians of more than 102,000 children and found that ADHD prevalence rates still varied widely between states. ("Mental Health in the United States: Prevalence of Diagnosis and Medication Treatment for Attetnion-Deficit/Hyperactivity Disorder—United States, 2003," *Centers for Disease Control and Prevention, Morbidity and Mortality Weekly Report*, Vol. 54 (34), pp. 842–47.

One 2005 study, furthermore, found that children living in upstate New York had about a tenfold higher chance of being given a stimulant prescription than similar children in New York City. (Marleen Radigan et al., "Medication Patterns for Attention-Deficit/Hyperactivity Disorder and Comorbid Psychiatric Conditions in a Low-Income Population," *Journal of Child and Adolescent Psychopharmacology*, Vol. 15 (1), 2005, pp. 44–56.)

72 At last count: In the 1990s, the gap was even greater. One 1999 study found it ranging between 9.4 percent in Georgia to 1.6 percent in Puerto Rico. Cited in Emily Arcia, Marcia C. Fernandez, and Marisela Jaquez, "Latina Mothers' Stances on Stimulant Medication: Complexity, Conflict, and Compromise," *Journal of Developmental & Behavioral Pediatrics*, Vol. 25 (5), October 2004, pp. 311–17.

There wasn't much standardization in how the disorder was being diagnosed or treated in the nineties. And some studies then indicated that kids who really didn't have the disorder were being inappropriately given meds. Researchers Adrian Angold and Jane Costello, for example, interviewed the parents of 1,422 children in the Smoky Mountains of North Carolina in the early and mid-1990s, and found that some children were indeed taking stimulants without having a valid ADHD diagnosis. Through their interviews, Angold and Costello diagnosed ADHD in 3.4 percent of the children, and found that an additional 2.8 percent qualified for the broader diagnosis of ADHD/NOS [not otherwise specified; i.e., some symptoms were present but the children didn't meet explicit criteria]—a total of 6.2 percent of the children. Yet, slightly over 7 percent of the children in the survey had received stimulants. Of the children taking stimulants, only 40 percent had received a formal ADHD diagnosis and almost 60 percent "never had parent-reported impairing ADHD symptoms of any sort," they noted. (Cited in Kalikow, p. 179.)

Columbia University psychiatrist Peter Jensen, on the other hand, surveyed 1,285 other children and parents nationwide in the late 1990s, and found a picture of undermedication. Only 12.5 percent of the children who met the criteria for ADHD in his study were being medicated, he reported. (Eliot Marshall, "Duke Study Faults Overuse of Stimulants for Children," *Science*, Vol. 289 (5480), August 2000, p. 721.)

Even in the Angold study, only 75 percent of the kids who met the formal diagnosis of ADHD actually took medication.

72 The really huge numbers . . . have never proven to be valid: "Although some children are being diagnosed as having ADHD with insufficient evaluation and in some cases stimulant medication is prescribed when treatment alternatives exist, there is little evidence of widespread overdiagnosis or misdiagnosis of ADHD or of widespread overprescription of methylphenidate [Ritalin] by physicians," the American Medical Association's Council on Scientific Affairs said, in the late 1990s, after the public panic over ADHD overdiagnosis and overtreatment led the AMA to review all the available studies on prescribing and diagnosing patterns of ADHD in children nationwide, along with Drug Enforcement Agency documents. L. S. Goldman et al., "Diagnosis and treatment of attention-deficit/hyperactivity disorder in children and adolescents," Council on Scientific Affairs, American Medical Association, published in *JAMA*, Vol. 279 (14), April 8, 1998, pp. 1100–7.

72 That a whole lot of kids are getting false ADHD diagnoses . . . hasn't held up: There are some indications that doctors have in recent years been doing a better job diagnosing ADHD in kids who really have it and treating those who really needed to be treated. This, at least, was the conclusion of a 2002 Mayo Clinic study, which followed a group of nearly six thousand children born between 1976 and 1982 in Rochester, New York, and, using survey questionnaires, school records, and medical records, divided them up into groups having "definite" ADHD (a clinical diagnosis plus at least one other kind of supporting documentation), "probable" ADHD (a clinical diagnosis but no other supporting documentation or no clinical diagnosis but two kinds of supporting documentation), "question-

able" ADHD (no clinical diagnosis, but at least one type of supporting documentation), and "not" ADHD. In the "definite" ADHD group, which comprised 7.4 percent of the children, 86.5 percent had been prescribed stimulant medication as treatment; in the group having "probable" ADHD, 40 percent had been prescribeda stimulant; in the "questionable" group, 6.6 percenthad received a prescription for a stimulant, and 0.2 percent of those in the "not ADHD" group had also received a prescription for meds.

William J. Barbaresi et al., "How Common Is Attention-Deficit/Hyperactivity Disorder?" *Archives of Pediatric and Adolescent Medicine*, Vol. 156, 2002, pp. 217–24.

72 Overuse and underuse of antidepressants: Some research has found antidepressants to be improperly used, given to mildy depressed children instead of the most afflicted, and given to children as young as age two, without any science to back up such use. The bottom line, child psychiatrist Kevin T. Kalikow concludes, in his excellent 2006 book, *Your Child in the Balance: An Insider's Guide for Parents to the Psychiatric Medication Dilemma,* is that "antidepressants are probably both under- and overprescribed: underprescribed to some patients with moderate to severe depression and overprescribed to others with less severe depression or in age groups or diagnostic categories for whom its benefit has not been proven": Kalikow, p. 183.

72 Childhood depression "among the least likely . . . to receive treatment": Brea L. Perry, Bernice A. Pescosolido, Jack K. Martin, Jane D. McLeod, and Peter S. Jensen, "Comparison of Public Attributions, Attitudes, and Stigma in Regard to Depression Among Children and Adults," *Psychiatric Services*, Vol. 58 (5), May 2007, pp. 632–35.

72 Just over half a million kids on atypicals: Carmen Moreno et al., "National Trends in the Outpatient Diagnosis and Treatment of Bipolar Disorder in Youth," *Archives of General Psychiatry*, Vol. 64 (9), September 2007, pp. 1032–39. Half a million to a million kids have been diagnosed as bipolar: Rosalie Greenberg, *Bipolar Kids: Helping Your Child Find Calm in the Mood Storm* (Cambridge, MA: Da Capo Press, 2007), p. ix.

The U.S. Department of Health and Human Services asserts that at least 750,000 children in the United States suffer from bipolar disorder. http://mentalhealth.samhsa.gov/publications/allpubs/CA-0006/default.asp#10.

And 60 *Minutes* reported in 2007 that nearly one million children had been diagnosed as bipolar. "What Killed Rebecca Riley?" CBS News, September 30, 2007.

81 Whenever they could, parents tried to stop medication: This is frequently the case. One 2005 study of a "high risk sample" of elementary school students screened for ADHD found that 35 percent of the children had received ADHD medications during a two-year period; about a third discontinued their treatment by the second year. Only 28 percent took advantage of school services and took their medications beyond the two-year period. Over a third of the children taking medication stopped its use within twelve months. The researchers found care for ADHD "remarkable for underuse and attrition of medical treatment, as well as poor linkage to relevant school services." (Regina Bussing et al., "Use and Persistence of Pharmacotherapy for Elementary School Students with Attention-Deficit/Hyperactivity Disorder," *Journal of Child and Adolescent Psychopharmacology* Vol. 15 (1), 2005, pp. 78–87.)

83 "We live the kind of life": Kristen, responding to "The Med Scare," *Domestic Disturbances*, nytimes.com, February 23, 2008.

84 70 to 80 percent of the time: NYU Child Study Center, "Facts About Children and Adolescents with ADHD," aboutourkids.org.

84 Up to 75 percent of parents: Emily Arcia, Marcia C. Fernandez, and Marisela Jaquez, "Latina Mothers' Stances on Stimulant Medication: Complexity, Conflict, and Compromise," *Journal of Developmental & Behavioral Pediatrics*, Vol. 25 (5), October 2004, pp. 311–17.

84 The fear of being prescribed medication: Susan dosReis, Matthew P. Mychailyszyn, MaryAnne Myers, and Anne W. Riley, "Coming to Terms with ADHD: How Urban African-American Families Come to Seek Care for Their Children," *Psychiatric Services*, Vol. 58 (5), May 2007, pp. 636–41.

85 "A beautiful, brilliant girl": "anna" response to Judith Warner, "Second Thoughts," nytimes.com, March 2, 2007.

87 Why parents cling to debunked ideas: Regina Bussing, Nancy E. Schoenberg, and Amy R. Perwien, "Knowledge and Information About ADHD: Evidence of Cultural Differences Among African-American and White Parents," *Social Science Medicine*, Vol. 46 (7), 1998, pp. 919–28, make this argument vis-à-vis African-American parents, but I've found it to be true for parents of all ethnic groups: "Parents may be particularly receptive to recommendations supporting a dietary etiology of ADHD," they write, "because this approach increases their perceived ability to control and manage child behavior symptoms." People continue to believe ADHD is caused by diet, though twenty years ago it was determined that it was not. Dr. Rachel Klein, for example, did a double-blind study to see if the Feingold

Diet—one free of all food additives—could be effective in treating children with ADHD. At the end, parents and doctors couldn't tell the children who'd been on the diet from others who hadn't. "Interview with Dr. Harold Koplewicz, founder and director of the New York University Child Study Center," washingtonpost.com, October 7, 2003.

87 "Messages" from caterpillars: Lisa Carver, "My Other Half," in Denise Brodey, ed., *The Elephant in the Playroom: Ordinary Parents Write Intimately and Honestly About the Extraordinary Highs and Heartbreaking Lows of Raising Kids with Special Needs* (New York: Hudson Street Press, 2007), p. 35.

88 "Quest for a cause": Perri Klass and Eileen Costello, *Quirky Kids: Understanding and Helping Your Child Who Doesn't Fit In—When to Worry and When Not to Worry* (New York: Ballantine, 2003), p. 68.

Chapter 5: Who, Exactly, Is Having Issues?

91 "'Here, take this pill'": Benedict Carey, "Parenting as Therapy for Child's Mental Disorders," *The New York Times*, December 22, 2006, p. A1.

92 "An ideal village": Response to "Second Thoughts," *The New York Times* online, March 1, 2007.

93 Inspiring headlines: "Parents Push the New Abnormal," USATODAY.com, October 1, 2006.

93 Parents don't like or want to use psychiatric drugs: See S. Hack and B. Chow, "Pediatric psychotropic medication compliance: a literature review and research-based suggestions for improving treatment compliance," *Journal of Child and Adolescent Psychopharmacology*, Vol. 11 (1), Spring, 2001, pp. 59–67. Also see: Helen Lazaratou et al., "Parental attitudes and opinions on the use of psychotropic medication in mental disorders of childhood," *Annals of General Psychiatry*, Vol. 6, November 2007, p. 32.

93 Many children end up being diagnosed as bipolar: Demitri and Janice Papolos, *The Bipolar Child* (New York: Broadway Books, 2002), p. xiv.

94 A damning portrait: Elizabeth J. Roberts, "A Rush to Medicate Young Minds," *The Washington Post*, October 8, 2006, p. B7.

94 A "hypothetical example": Roy Richard Grinker, *Unstrange Minds: Remapping the World of Autism* (New York: Basic Books, 2007), p. 135.

96 Doctors who'd been very vocal, in print: Lawrence H. Diller writes that many of

the kids caught up in the culture of diagnosis are primarily victims of our sick culture, "Tom Sawyers and Pippi Longstockings who are not meeting the expectations for children in modern-day America," in *The Last Normal Child: Essays on the Intersection of Kids, Culture, and Psychiatric Drugs* (Westport: Praeger, 2006), p. 36.

96 "I, in my role as specialist": Ibid., p. 14.

97 "Virtually all parents": "Dave G.," response to Judith Warner, "Ritalin Wars," nytimes.com, November 17, 2007.

98 One Bay Area educational psychologist: C. W. Nevius, "A Slippery Slope: The New Parental Ethics Teach All the Wrong Life Lessons," *The San Francisco Chronicle*, October 19, 2003.

98 Horseback riding and personal trainers: Alison Leigh Cowan, "In an Affluent Town, Parents and Schools Clash Over Special Education," *The New York Times*, April 24, 2005.

98 "Educational scam": Mary Eberstadt, *Home-Alone America: The Hidden Toll of Day Care, Behavioral Drugs, and Other Parent Substitutes* (New York: Sentinel, 2004), p. 71.

99 Up to $150,000 a year: Kathleen Carroll, "Special Ed's Costs Endanger Other Programs," NorthJersey.com, February 24, 2008.

99 Washington, D.C., parents . . . learned: Dan Keating and V. Dion Haynes, "Special-Ed Tuition a Growing Drain on D.C.," *The Washington Post*, June 5, 2006, p. A1.

100 Tom Freston: Joseph Berger, "Fighting Over When Public Should Pay Private Tuition for Disabled," *The New York Times*, March 21, 2007.

100 New York City education officials: Ibid.

100 The most competitive . . . The most affluent: Mary Eberstadt, in *Home-Alone America*, p. 70 ff, writes, "It is the country's most exclusive and competitive schools that register the highest rates of learning disability." She quotes Michael Scott Moore in a 2000 essay for *Salon*, saying that while nationwide only 1.9 percent of students get a "special accommodation" for the SAT, in some New England prep schools and in wealthy California districts the number rises to nearly 10 percent. She notes that Arthur Levine, president of Teachers College, Columbia, reported in 2000 that 36 percent of kindergarteners at the exclusive Dalton School in Manhattan had learning problems. She also notes that the *Los Angeles Times* found that "students receiving special treatments are concentrated in the wealthiest communities and that students enrolled in private prep schools are two to five times as likely to get extended time on the SAT." But Eberstadt's

information and interpretations have to be taken with a grain of salt. Her Dalton example is highly misleading, as it's a statistic derived from a period when the school had embarked upon a (short-lived) experiment with running a remedial program for students with learning issues. This program was long gone by 2000, when Levine's op-ed ran in the *Times*. See Diane Ravitch and Joseph P. Viteritti, eds, *City Schools: Lessons from New York* (Baltimore: Johns Hopkins University Press, 2000), p. 226.

101 Legal and financial hurdles: Daniel Golden, "Staying the Course," *The Wall Street Journal*, July 24, 2007.

101 The wealthiest and most sophisticated: Judith Sealander, *The Failed Century of the Child: Governing America's Young in the Twentieth Century* (Cambridge: Cambridge University Press, 2003), p. 280 ff.

101 A nonworking spouse: Ibid.

104 In Houston: Jennifer Radcliffe, "Schools Fail to Meet Law on Dyslexia," *The Houston Chronicle*, June 18, 2007.

105 In Georgia: Bridget Gutierrez, "Vouchers for Disabled Students Popular but Limited," *The Atlanta Journal-Constitution*, December 17, 2007.

105 On Long Island: John Hildebrand, "Gaps Seen in Communities' Student Autism Services," Newsday.com, January 16, 2008.

105 In Massachusetts: Pamela White, "Autism Epidemic," *Boulder Weekly*, April 12, 2007.

106 In Colorado: Ibid.

106 "From the couch to the crib": Elizabeth Bernstein, "Sending the Baby to a Shrink," *The Wall Street Journal*, October 24, 2006, p. D1.

106 Only 5 to 7 percent: *Blueprint for Change: Research on Child and Adolescent Mental Health*, Report of the National Advisory Mental Health Council Workgroup on Child and Adolescent Mental Health Intervention Development and Deployment, Washington, D.C., May 2001, p. 34.

106 70 percent: American Academy of Pediatrics website, www.aap.org/commpeds/dochs/mentalhealth/index.cfm. The U.S. Department of Health and Human Services says that two-thirds of children with mental health problems are not getting help. NYU Child Study Center says only one out of every five children with a psychiatric disorder gets treatment. (Interview with Harold Koplewicz, April 2, 2008; www.aboutourkids.org.)

106 Fewer than 25 percent: Carlos Blanco et al., "Mental Health of College Students and Their Non-College-Attending Peers: Results from the National Epidemio-

logic Study on Alcohol and Related Conditions," *Archives of General Psychiatry*, Vol. 65 (12), 2008, pp. 1429–37.

106 Only 5 percent: Author interview with Mark Olfson, April 21, 2008.

106 Only 9 percent: Patricia Alex, "Students with Mental Troubles on Rise," *The Record*, June 25, 2007.

107 Three to six weeks: Richard C. Paddock, "Suicides a Symptom of Larger UC Crisis," *Los Angeles Times*, May 23, 2007.

107 Deficiencies are "staggering": *Blueprint for Change*, p. 36.

107 About seven thousand: Author interview with Kristin Kroeger Ptakowski, Senior Deputy Executive Director, Director of Government Affairs and Clincal Practice, the American Academy of Child and Adolescent Psychiatry, Feb. 19, 2009.

107 Pediatricians fail to recognize and refer kids: John V. Campo, "Addressing the Interface Between Pediatrics and Psychiatry," *Psychiatric Times*, September 1, 2004, p. 40.

107 In North Carolina: Lidia Wasowicz, "Ped Med: Young Minds Under Attack," United Press International, January 9, 2006.

107 An eight-to-twelve minute consultation: "National Survey of Pediatricians Says Time Restraints Affect Quality of Medical Care for Children," U.S. Newswire, February 4, 2003.

108 Families fail to follow up: John V. Campo, "Addressing the Interface Between Pediatrics and Psychiatry," *Psychiatric Times*, September 1, 2004, p. 40.

108 Most parents believe more strongly in therapy: Helen Lazaratou et al., "Parental Attitudes and Opinions on the use of Psychotropic Medication in Mental Disorders of Childhood," *Annals of General Psychiatry*, Vol. 6, November, 2007, p. 32.

108 More than half of all outpatient services: *Blueprint for Change*, p. 34. Because of low reimbursement rates for talk therapy and no reimbursement for follow-up time with parents and schools, a Connecticut survey in 2007 showed that fully half of the state's child psychiatrists would no longer accept insurance and were making patients pay out of pocket. See William Hathaway, "Kids' Mental Health Care Imperiled," *The Hartford Courant*, April 13, 2007. Children without health insurance are, not surprisingly, the group least likely to get mental health services at all. (*Blueprint*, p. 34).

108 A veneer of "well-being": Suniya Luthar and Shawn J. Latendresse, "Children of the Affluent: Challenges to Well-Being," *Current Directions in Psychological Science*, Vol. 14, February 2005, p. 49.

108 Levine concludes: Madeline Levine, *The Price of Privilege: How Parental Pressure and*

Material Advantage Are Creating a Generation of Disconnected and Unhappy Kids (New York: HarperCollins, 2006), p. 26.

108 African-American children less likely to be diagnosed: Jack Stevens, Jeffrey S. Harman, and Kelly J. Kelleher, "Race/Ethnicity and Insurance Status as Factors Associated with ADHD Treatment Patterns," *Journal of Child and Adolescent Psychopharmacology*, Vol. 15 (1), 2005, pp. 88–96.

108 Perception that black children are being singled out: Regina Bussing, Nancy E. Schoenberg, and Amy R. Perwien, "Knowledge and Information About ADHD: Evidence of Cultural Differences Among African-American and White Parents," *Social Science Medicine*, Vol. 46 (7), 1998, pp. 919–28.

108 Black children are far less likely than white kids to take medication: Jack Stevens, Jeffrey S. Harman, and Kelly J. Kelleher, "Race/Ethnicity and Insurance Status as Factors Associated with ADHD Treatment Patterns," *Journal of Child and Adolescent Psychopharmacology*, Vol. 15 (1), 2005, pp. 88–96.

108 One 2003 study: Laurel K. Leslie, Jill Weckerly, John Landsverk, Richard L. Hough, Michael S. Hurlburt, and Patricia A. Wood, "Racial/Ethnic Differences in the Use of Psychotropic Medication in High-Risk Children and Adolescents," *Journal of the American Academy of Child & Adolescent Psychiatry*, Vol. 42 (23) December 2003, pp. 1433–42.

109 Minority children suffer disproportionately: *Blueprint*, p. 21 ff.

109 Black children viewed as "bad": Bussing, Schoenberg, and Perwien, "Knowledge and Information about ADHD: Evidence of Cultural Differences Among African–American and White Parents," pp. 919–928.

109 Black students suspended and expelled: Howard Witt, "School Discipline Tougher on African Americans," *Chicago Tribune*, September 25, 2007.

110 "Provider bias": "Provider biases regarding explanations for behavioral problems and viable treatment options in children from different racial/ethnic backgrounds would also hypothetically affect the quality of care received. . . . Different beliefs about the causes of illness and the acceptability of and expectation for treatment by patients of varied cultural backgrounds have been shown to alter diagnostic and treatment patterns for psychiatric disorders," say Laurel K. Leslie, Jill Weckerly, John Landsverk, Richard L. Hough, Michael S. Hurlburt, and Patricia A. Wood in "Racial/Ethnic Differences in the Use of Psychotropic Medication in High-Risk Children and Adolescents," *Journal of the American Academy of Child & Adolescent Psychiatry*, Vol. 42 (23) December 2003, pp. 1433–42.

110 Distrust of psychologists and psychiatrists: Bussing, Schoenberg, and Perwien,

"Knowledge and Information about ADHD: Evidence of Cultural Differences Among African-American and White Parents," pp. 919–28.

111 "Expert" beliefs about genetic inferiority: Jason Schnittker, Jeremy Freese, and Brian Powell, "Nature, Nurture, Neither, Nor: Black-White Differences in Beliefs About the Causes and Appropriate Treatment of Mental Illness," *Social Forces*, Vol. 78 (3), March 2000, pp. 1101–30.

111 Psychologists as "impersonal": Vetta L. Sanders Thompson, Anita Bazile, and Maysa Akbar, "African Americans' Perceptions of Psychotherapy and Psychotherapists," *Professional Psychology: Research and Practice*, Vol. 35 (10), pp. 19–26.

112 "Finger-pointing": James P. Guevara, Chris Feudtner, Daniel Romer, Thomas Power, Ricardo Eiraldi, Snejana Nitianova, Aracely Rosales, Janet Ohene-Frempong, and Donald F. Schwarz, "Fragmented Care for Inner-City Minority Children with Attention-Deficit/Hyperactivity Disorder," *Pediatrics*, Vol. 116 (4), October 2005, pp. 512–17.

113 "Fail up": Christopher Bellonci, Author interview. February 19, 2009.

113 In Virginia: "Improving the Quality of Health Care for Mental and Substance-Use Conditions," a report of the Institute of Medicine, 2006.

114 "Why on God's green earth": Matthew Hansen and Karyn Spencer, "Safe Haven Meant Kids Finally Got Right Help," Omaha.com, February 1, 2009.

Chapter 6: "B-a-d" Children, Worse Parents (and Even Worse Doctors)

118 "Rudest in history": Susan Gregory Thomas, "Today's Tykes: Secure Kids or Rudest in History?" msnbc.com, May 6, 2009.

118 Only 9 percent of respondents: Judith Warner, "Kids Gone Wild," *The New York Times*, November 27, 2005, Week in Review, p. 1.

118 Toddlers expelled from preschool: In May 2005, a Yale University Child Center study found that more than 5,000 children per year were being asked to leave state-financed preschools, a rate three times higher than public school students in K-12. See W. S. Gilliam, "Prekindergarteners left behind: Expulsion rates in state prekindergarten systems," New Haven, CT: Yale University Child Study Center, 2005.

118 Schoolchildren so undisciplined: Claudia Wallis, "Does Kindergarten Need Cops?" *Time*, December 15, 2003, p. 52.

118 More than one in three teachers: Warner, "Kids Gone Wild."

119 "B-a-d" kids: Wallis, "Does Kindergarten Need Cops?" p. 52.

119 A Chicago café owner: Jodi Wilgoren, "At Center of a Clash, Rowdy Children in Coffee Shops," *The New York Times*, November 9, 2005, p. A12.

119 "Disruptive urchins": John Rosemond, "Restaurant No Place for Playground Antics," washingtontimes.com, November 5, 2005.

119 They can't say no: Peg Tyre, "The Power of No," *Newsweek*, September 13, 2004, p. 42.

119 They outsource etiquette: CBS News, "More Parents Outsourcing Etiquette," May 12, 2005.

120 Parent coaches: Pam Belluck, "With Mayhem at Home, They Call a Parent Coach," *The New York Times*, March 13, 2005, p. A1.

120 Experts script them: Tyre, "The Power of No," p. 42.

120 Parents screaming at, assaulting coaches: Nancy Gibbs, "Parents Behaving Badly," *Time*, February 21, 2005, p. 40.

120 More than half of educators: Warner, "Kids Gone Wild."

120 "New class of bullies": Sarah Carr, "Parents Are New Class of Bullies," *Milwaukee Journal Sentinel*, May 20, 2006.

121 Some 40 percent of children: Rahul K. Parikh, "Growth Hormones for Kids," Salon.com, October 31, 2008.

121 "As some become taller": Michael J. Sandel, "The Case against Perfection," *The Atlantic Monthly*, April 1, 2004, p. 50.

122 Girls as young as nine: Linda A. Johnson, "More Girls Using Steroids, Studies Say," Associated Press, April 26, 2005.

122 One in eight boys: Elizabeth Weise, "Adolescents Bulk Up Their Bodies," *USA Today*, August 22, 2005.

122 More than 90 percent: This is a survey of 25,000 high school students from 2001 to 2008 by Dr. Donald McCabe of Rutgers University. Cited in Maura J. Casey, "Digging Out Roots of Cheating in High School," *The New York Times*, October 13, 2008.

122 "Nothing shocks us": Jodi S. Cohen, "Students Add Sabotage to College-Entry Arsenal," *Chicago Tribune*, October 20, 2008.

123 "Toddlerhood in perpetuity": John Rosemond and Bose Ravenel, *The Diseasing of America's Children* (Nashville, TN:Thomas Nelson, 2008), p. 161.

123 The "pursuit of better-behaved . . . children": *Beyond Therapy: Biotechnology and*

the Pursuit of Happiness, A Report by the President's Council on Bioethics, Washington, D.C., October 15, 2003, p. 27.

124 *Frontline*'s highly disturbing documentary: "The Medicated Child," *Frontline*, January 8, 2008.

125 ADHD meds as cheating aid: Colin MeGill, "Adderall: The Steroids of Intellect," *The Daily Campus*, May 11, 2004.

125 Drugs as SAT score-booster: Nicholas Zamiska, "Pressed to Do Well on Admissions Tests, Students Take Drugs," *The Wall Street Journal*, November 8, 2004.

125 "'Brother's little helper'": Harry Jaffe and Alex Chip, "Got Any Smart Pills?" *Washingtonian*, January 2006, p. 41.

126 "Popular performance aid": Unmesh Kher, "Can You Find Concentration in a Bottle?" *Time*, January 16, 2006, p. 98.

126 Even *professors*: Sahakian and Morein-Zamir, "Professor's Little Helper," *Nature*, Vol. 450, December 20, 2007 pp. 1157–59.

126 A bioethicist: Karen Kaplan, "They're Bulking Up Mentally," *Los Angeles Times*, December 20, 2007, p. A1.

127 "Academics don't get paid very much": Gardiner Harris, Benedict Carey, and Janet Roberts, "Psychiatrists, Troubled Children and Drug Industry's Role," *The New York Times*, May 10, 2007, p. A1.

127 "Too cozy relationships": http://www.senate.gov/~finance/press/Gpress/2005/prg092006.pdf

127 DelBello had claimed about $100,00: Gardiner Harris, "Lawmaker Calls for Registry of Drug Firms Paying Doctors," *The New York Times*, August 4, 2007. And Benedict Carey and Gardiner Harris, "Psychiatric Association Faces Senate Scrutiny Over Drug Industry Ties," *The New York Times*, July 12, 2008, p. A13.

128 Biederman had earned at least $1.6 million: Gardiner Harris and Benedict Carey, "Researchers Fail to Reveal Full Drug Pay," *The New York Times*, June 8, 2008.

128 Thirty percent of its $62.5 million: Carey and Harris, "Psychiatric Association Faces Senate Scrutiny Over Drug Industry Ties," p. A13. And Ed Silverman, "Grassley Probes Psychiatrists Over Ties to Pharma," Pharmalot.com, July 11, 2008.

128 Dr. Charles B. Nemeroff . . . had failed to report: Gardiner Harris, "Top Psychiatrist Didn't Report Drug Makers' Pay," *The New York Times*, October 3, 2008.

128 "I regret the failure of full disclosure": "Emory Announces Actions Following Investigation," Emory University Press Release, December 22, 2008.

128 DelBello eventually complained: Doug Lederman, "Scrutiny of Researcher-Industry Ties," *Inside Higher Education*, August 6, 2007.

128 Schatzberg told *The New York Times*: Benedict Carey and Gardiner Harris, "Psychiatric Group Ceases Scrutiny Over Drug Industry Ties," *The New York Times*, July 12, 2008.

129 The APA objected: Author interview with Paul Thacker in Senator Grassley's office.

129 Conflicts . . . "permeate": Marcia Angell, "Industry-Sponsored Clinical Research: A Broken System," *JAMA*, Vol. 300, No. 9, 2008, pp. 1069–71.

129 About two-thirds of academic research centers: Ibid.

130 97 percent of third-year medical students: Author interview with Eric Campbell, associate professor of medicine, at the Institute for Health Policy, Massachusetts General Hospital and Harvard Medical School, who studies the relationship between academia and industry, November 5, 2008.

130 Cardiologists: Author interview with Paul Thacker in Senator Grassley's office.

131 Orthopedic surgeons: David Armstrong, "Lawsuit Says Medtronic Gave Doctors Array of Perks," wsj.com, September 25, 2008.

131 Such good drama: Cited in Ed Silverman, "Boston Legal: TV Drama Or Reality Show?" Pharmalot.com, October 29, 2008.

131 Biederman research criticized: Author interviews with Marcia Angell and news reports.

131 Virtually no research: By 2006, there were still only a "handful" of small studies testing the powerful new class of antipsychotics (none of which had at that point been approved for pediatric use) on children and teens. Benedict Carey, "Use of Antipsychotics by Young People in U.S. Rose Fivefold in Decade, Researchers Report," *The New York Times*, June 6, 2006.

132 FDA data from 2000 to 2004: Marilyn Elias, "New Antipsychotic Drugs Carry Risks for Children," *USA Today*, May 2, 2006.

132 In 2006, antipsychotics were the "primary suspect": Gardiner Harris, Benedict Carey, and Janet Roberts, "Psychiatrists, Children, and Drug Industry's Role," *The New York Times*, May 10, 2007, p. A1.

132 Tiny fraction: so said, among others, former FDA Commissioner Dr. Mark B. McClellan, in "A Shot at Making Drugs Safer," *Business Week*, May 21, 2007.

132 "Medicopharmaceutical industrial complex": The phrase is from Richard DeGrandpre, *The Cult of Pharmacology: How America Became the World's Most Troubled Drug Culture* (Durham: Duke University Press, 2006), p. 170.

132 E-mails emerged: Gardiner Harris, "Research Center Tied to Drug Company," *The New York Times*, November 25, 2008.

133 Biederman defended himself: Liz Kowalczyk, "Psychiatrist Responds to Charges," *The Boston Globe*, December 6, 2008.

133 The doctor agreed: Pam Belluck, "Child Psychiatrist to Curtail Industry-Financed Activities," *The New York Times*, December 31, 2008.

133 Psychiatrists were overrepresented: See State of Vermont, Office of the Attorney General, news release, July 8, 2008.

133 When *The New York Times* in May 2007, analyzed records: Harris, Carey, and Roberts, "Psychiatrists, Troubled Children, and Drug Industry's Role," p. A1.

134 The MTA study: Peter S. Jensen et al., "3-Year Follow-up of the NIMH MTA Study," *Journal of the American Academy of Child & Adolescent Psychiatry*, Vol. 46 (8), August 2007, pp. 988–1000.

135 Suppressing information about side effects: Wayne Kondro and Barbara Sibbald, "Drug Company Experts Advised Staff to Withhold Data About SSRI Use in Children," *Canadian Medical Association Journal*, Vol. 170 (5), March 2, 2004, p. 783.

135 Bringing new drugs to market that are no more effective: "Newer Antipsychotics No Better Than Older Drug in Treating Child and Adolescent Schizophrenia," National Institute of Mental Health Press Release, September 15, 2008.

135 Encouraging physicians: Alex Berenson, "Drug Files Show Maker Promoted Unapproved Use," *The New York Times*, December 18, 2006, p. A1.

135 60 percent of those clinical studies: Shannon Brownlee, "Doctors Without Borders: Why You Can't Trust Medical Journals Anymore," *The Washington Monthly*, April 2004.

136 About a third of the drugs: Joseph Deveaugh-Geiss et al., "Child and Adolescent Psychopharmacology in the New Millennium: A Workshop for Academia, Industry, and Government," *Journal of the American Academy of Child & Adolescent Psychiatry*, Vol. 45 (3), March 2006, pp. 261–70.

136 Paxil "generally well tolerated": Kondro and Sibbald, "Drug Company Experts Advised Staff to Withhold Data About SSRI Use in Children," p. 783.

137 'Drugs are often widely prescribed": Deveaugh-Geiss et al., "Child and Adolescent Psychopharmacology in the New Millennium: A Workshop for Academia, Industry, and Government," pp. 261–70.

137 A number of state attorneys general: Ed Silverman, "J&J Sued by Arkansas Over Risperdal Marketing," Pharmalot.com, November 20, 2007. And author interview with Camp Bailey, lawyer with Bailey Perrin Bailey in Houston.

137 Janssen alone was accused: Margaret Cronin Fisk and David Voreacos, "J&J Unit Marketed Risperdal Drug Off-Label, Former Workers Say," Bloomberg News, March 7, 2009.

137 Although Risperdal has no role in treating ADHD . . . 16 percent of pediatric users taking it: Judith Warner, "Tough Choices for Tough Children," nytimes.com, November 20, 2008.

137 Forest Laboratories charged with paying kickbacks to doctors: All in violation of federal anti-kickback laws and in violation of Medicaid policy, which does not normally cover off-label uses of drugs unless the use is for a medically accepted indication. Barry Meier and Benedict Carey, "Drug Maker Is Accused of Fraud," *The New York Times*, February 26, 2009. And "United States Files Complaint Against Forest Laboratories for Allegedly Violating the False Claims Act," U.S. Department of Justice, Office of Public Affairs Press Release, February 25, 2009.

138 "If you can define": Vince Parry, "The Art of Branding a Condition," *Medical Marketing and Media*, May 2003, Vol 38 (5), p. 43.

138 Even industry leaders: Troyen A. Brennan et al., "Sunshine Laws and the Pharmaceutical Industry," *JAMA*, Vol. 297, 2007, pp. 1255–57.

138 By 2009, there were signs that doctors were growing far more cautious: Prescriptions for psychiatric drugs for children under ten increased 3.5 percent in 2008, *The Wall Street Journal* reported, whereas, between 2002 and 2007, they rose 44.6 percent. There was also a 1 percent drop in prescriptions for children under age seven. See David Armstrong, "Children's Use of Psychiatric Drugs Begins to Decelerate," *The Wall Street Journal*, May 18, 2009.

139 The Food and Drug Administration . . . has become severely compromised: Howard Markel, "Why America Needs a Strong FDA," *JAMA*, Vol. 294, No. 19, November 16, 2005, pp. 2489–91.

139 "Although these individuals are supposed to recuse themselves": Angell, "Industry-Sponsored Clinical Research: A Broken System," pp. 1069–71.

140 Grassley . . . accused the agency of outright collusion: Both from letter from Senator Charles E. Grassley to FDA Commissioner Andrew C. von Eschenbach, "RE: Off-Label Promotion of Drugs," April 21, 2008.

140 Dr. Andrew Mosholder: Shankar Vedantam, "FDA Told Its Analyst to Censor Data on Antidepressants," *The Washington Post*, September 24, 2004, p. A8, and Gardiner Harris, "Expert Kept from Speaking at Antidepressant Hearing," *The New York Times*, Friday, April 16, 2004.

140 82 Percent of Americans . . . and another 80 percent: Beckey Bright, "Americans Growing Less Confident In FDA's Job on Safety, Poll Shows," *The Wall Street Journal*, May 24, 2006.

141 The National Institutes of Health were forced to turn themselves inside out: Marcia Angell, *The Truth About the Drug Companies* (New York: Random House, 2004), pp. 104–5.

141 The NIH adopted strict new ethics rules: Gardiner Harris, "Agency Scientists Divided Over Ethics Ban on Consulting," *The New York Times*, February 2, 2005.

142 "Doctors are more stigmatized than the illness": Author interview with Thomas Insel, November 2008.

143 "The hubris of drug companies": Judith Warner, "Diagnosis: Greed," nytimes .com, October 9, 2008.

Chapter 7: Stuck in the Cuckoo's Nest

145 "An unparalleled tragedy": Eric G. Wilson, *Against Happiness* (New York: Farrar, Straus and Giroux, 2008), p. 149.

146 "Sudden extinction of the creative impulse": Ibid., p. 5.

146 "The sad consequence": Christopher Lane, *Shyness: How Normal Behavior Became a Sickness* (New Haven: Yale University Press, 2007), p. 8.

146 "Proof that one is alive": Charles Barber, *Comfortably Numb: How Psychiatry Is Medicating a Nation* (New York: Pantheon Books, 2008). "Medicated American" is p. 100, other quote p. 217.

146 *The Medicalization of Society . . . The Loss of Sadness:* Also see, from a bit earlier, sociologist Allan V. Horwitz's *Creating Mental Illness,* and journalist Ray Moynihan and policy researcher Alan Cassels's *Selling Sickness: How the World's Biggest Pharmaceutical Companies Are Turning Us All into Patients.* It's worth noting that Horwitz and Wakefield's is actually not against psychiatry per se, and makes a very convincing case for diagnostic reforms that would refine and improve the practice of the profession.

146 "'We called them *boys*'": Lane, p. 3.

147 "Bright and ambitious people": Gary Greenberg, "Manufacturing Depression: A Journey into the Economy of Melancholy," *Harper's*, May 1, 2007, p. 35.

147 "Political sedatives": Frederick C. Crews, "Talking Back to Prozac," *The New York Review of Books*, Vol. 54 (19), December 6, 2007.

147 "The arbiter of normality": Allan Horwitz, quoted in Shankar Vedantam, "Criteria for Depression Are Too Broad, Researchers Say," *The Washington Post*, April 3, 2007, p. A2.

147 "Changing what it means to be human": Ray Moynihan and Alan Cassels, *Selling Sickness: How the World's Biggest Pharmaceutical Companies Are Turning Us All Into Patients* (New York: Nation Books, 2005), p. x.

147 "How can we generalize normal?": Kevin M, responding to "Second Thoughts," nytimes.com., March 1, 2007.

148 "An enhanced ability": *Beyond Therapy: Biotechnology and the Pursuit of Happiness*, A Report by the President's Council on Bioethics, Washington, D.C., October 15, 2003, p. 89–90.

148 About 10 percent of Americans: Mark Olfson and Steven C. Marcus, "National Patterns in Anti-Depressant Medication Treatment," *Archives of General Psychiatry*, Vol. 66 (8), August 2009, p. 848.

148 It's inevitable: Allan V. Horwitz and Jerome C. Wakefield convincingly argue in *The Loss of Sadness* that *DSM-IV* criteria for depression do not explicitly enough distinguish between "normal sadness and depressive disorder" (p. 6). (Even Robert Spitzer, the "father" of the *DSM-III* admits, in a forward to Horwitz and Wakefield's book, that the criteria ought, perhaps, to be refined: "It should be noted that at the time the diagnostic criteria for depression were originally developed, they were intended for research samples in which it was a reasonable assumption that the patients were disordered. The authors argue that, when those same diagnostic criteria that contain no reference to context are used in community epidemiological studies and screening of the general population, large numbers of people who are having normal human responses to various stressors are mistakenly diagnosed as disordered. The researchers who have conducted the major epidemiological studies over the past two decades have totally ignored the problem." Spitzer, however, says he would still cast a wider net than Horwitz and Wakefield do, in identifying who ought to qualify for actual treatment.) And I wonder if the critique of epidemiological studies—which generate artificially high incidence rates for depression and other mental illnesses, to the delight of the pharmaceutical industry—really does carry over to office practice. After all, the people presenting in a doctor's office asking for Prozac (or being diagnosed as depressed on the spot) are not *necessarily* representatives of a general population sample. They perhaps conform more closely to the population Spitzer describes, where there's a "reasonable assumption" of actual disorder.

148 Mental disorders in adults are common and tend to go untreated: Just sticking with disorders treated by antidepressants: According to the National Institute of Mental Health, major depressive disorder (severe depression) affects 14.8 million adults over age eighteen in the U.S. each year, or 6.7 percent of the adult population. Another 1.5 percent of people suffer from chronic mild depression, or dysthymic disorder. Slightly over 18 percent of the over-eighteen population suffers from an anxiety disorder in any given year. Even if you assume that, because of the survey problems discussed by Horwitz and Wakefield (and many others), these numbers are somewhat inflated, they still indicate that antidepressant use is not, in fact, out of line with the prevalence of depression and anxiety in the population. http://www.nimh.nih.gov/health/publications/the-numbers-count-mental-disorders-in-america/index.shtml.

149 Barber . . . admits as much: Barber, p. xvi.

149 "Prozac in the Washington water supply": Author interview with Thomas Insel, November, 2008.

149 Treatment guidelines: "Use of Drugs to Treat Depression: Guidelines from the American College of Physicians," *Annals of Internal Medicine, Summaries for Patients,* Vol. 149 (10), November 18, 2008, pp. I–56.

149 "Cosmetic psychopharmacology": Peter D. Kramer, *Listening to Prozac: A Psychiatrist Explores Antidepressant Drugs and the Remaking of the Self* (New York: Viking, 1993), p. 15.

150 "Better than well": Ibid., p. x.

150 "People were taking my worries": Peter D. Kramer, in "The Truth About Prozac: An Exchange," nybooks.com, Vol. 55 (2), February 14, 2008.

151 "Biomedical social control leadership": Peter R. Breggin and Ginger Ross Breggin, *The War Against Children* (New York: St. Martin's, 1994), p. 6.

151 "Their losses made me personally aware": Lawrence H. Diller, *The Last Normal Child: Essays on the Intersection of Kids, Culture, and Psychiatric Drugs* (Westport: Praeger, 2006), p. 178.

153 "It is only the choice": Joanne Greenberg, *I Never Promised You a Rose Garden* (New York: Signet, 1964), p. 110.

153 "Pseudomedical form of social control": Thomas Szasz, quoted in Maggie Scarf, "Normality Is a Square Circle or a Four-Sided Triangle," *The New York Times Magazine*, October 3, 1971.

153 "There can be no such thing": Thomas Szasz, "Mental Illness: A Metaphorical Disease" (adapted from "Mental Illness as a Metaphor," *Nature*, Vol. 242 [5396],

March 30, 1973, pp. 305–7), in *The Medicalization of Everyday Life: Selected Essays* (Syracuse: Syracuse University Press), 2007, p. 4.

154 "Dedicating herself to adjustment": Ken Kesey, *One Flew Over the Cuckoo's Nest* (New York: Penguin, 2002), p. 25.

154 "A bitch and a buzzard": Ibid., p. 54.

155 He'd participated in government sponsored experiments: Robert Faggen, Introduction to *One Flew Over the Cuckoo's Nest* (New York: Penguin, 2002).

156 Window signs for Miltown: Jonathan Michel Metzel, *Prozac on the Couch: Prescribing Gender in the Era of Wonder Drugs* (Durham: Duke University Press, 2003), p. 73.

156 "Miltown-by-the-sea": Andrea Tone, *The Age of Anxiety: A History of America's Turbulent Affair with Tranquilizers* (New York: Basic Books, 2008), p. 55.

156 17 percent of people . . . and 30 percent reported: Gerald L. Klerman, "Psychotropic Hedonism vs. Pharmacological Calvinism," *The Hastings Center Report*, Vol. 2 (4), September, 1972, pp. 1–3.

156 Almost one woman in four and one man in ten: Peter D. Kramer, "Prozac Nation?" *Slate*, February 11, 2008. Shorter, p. 319, says one-fifth of women and one in thirteen men were using minor tranquilizers and sedatives.

156 "Refined form of lobotomy": David Healy, *The Creation of Psychopharmacology* (Cambridge: Harvard University Press, 2002), p. 134.

156 Valium and Miltown, disproportionately prescribed to women: Allan V. Horwitz and Jerome C. Wakefield, *The Loss of Sadness: How Psychiatry Transformed Normal Sorrow into Depressive Disorder* (New York: Oxford University Press, 2007), p. 180.

156 False schizophrenia diagnosis of Joanne Greenberg: Psychiatrists Remi Cadoret and Carol North, reanalyzing her case using *DSM-III* criteria in the *Archives of General Psychiatry* in 1981, stated that Greenberg had not been schizophrenic at all, but most likely suffering from depression, which could have remitted on its own or been helped with therapy. (Dava Sobel, "Schizophrenia in Popular Books: A Study Finds Too Much Hope," *The New York Times*, February 17, 1981.) Colleagues of Fromm-Reichmann also doubted the diagnosis, see Mari Jo Buhle, "Curing the Incurable," *The Women's Review of Books*, May 1, 2001, p. 12.

157 "Assaultive and belligerent?": Jonathan Michel Metzl's *Prozac on the Couch: Prescribing Gender in the Era of Wonder Drugs* (Durham: Duke University Press, 2003) has a wonderful gallery of drug advertisements over the decades. The Haldol ad appears on p. 30.

157 "Largely arbitrary": Herb Kutchins and Stuart A. Kirk, *Making Us Crazy: DSM:*

The Psychiatric Bible and the Creation of Mental Disorders (New York: The Free Press, 1997), p. 27.

157 "Obviously, those suffering" Wilson, p. 149.

158 "Laid-back, Southern aesthetic": Carl Elliott, *Better Than Well: American Medicine Meets the American Dream* (New York: W. W. Norton and Co., 2003), p. 250.

159 "Indigo children": John Leland, "Are They Here to Save the World?" *The New York Times*, January 12, 2006. And see, most recently, Lee Caroll and Jan Tober, *The Indigo Children Ten Years Later* (Carlsbad, CA: Hay House, 2009).

159 Brandenn Bremmer: Eric Konigsberg, "Prairie Fire: The Life and Death of a Prodigy," *The New Yorker*, January 16, 2006.

160 Sex offender: J. E. Wantz refers to himself as such in http://www.annefrank.com/prison-diary-program/excerpts-september-2008/.

160 "Have I been cheating myself": J. E. Wantz, "Feeling(s) Cheated," PEN.org, June 2007.

161 "The vogue for identifying autism": Michael Fitzpatrick, "The Trouble with Autism-Lit," spiked-online.com, July 21, 2006.

162 "Sweet, dreamy boy": Ann Bauer, "The Monster Inside My Son," Salon.com, March 26, 2009.

163 Gardiner Harris had written: Gardiner Harris, "Use of Antipsychotics in Children Is Criticized," *The New York Times*, November 18, 2008.

165 "Evidence aside": Author interview with Peter Kramer, February 13, 2008.

165 "Pharmacological Calvinism": Klerman, "Psychotropic Hedonism vs. Pharmacological Calvinism," pp. 1–3.

167 "The way neurochemicals tell stories": Kramer, *Listening to Prozac*, p. 21.

167 Symptom management . . . new and better ways of living: Here is a nice way of making clear the distinction between what the public believes—that there are "causes" of mental illness that stem from experience and that medication is a "quick fix" remedy that doesn't get at root causes the way that therapy would—and what psychiatrists now believe: "Many psychiatrists are skeptical about the validity of a causal approach to psychotherapy and believe that the etiology of most psychiatric disorders is largely unknown—though they expect extensive, genetic, epidemiologic, and neurobiologic research to ultimately identify important causal factors." But they do believe in therapy, just not therapy as a means of uncovering the *causes* of psychiatric disorders; rather as a way to help the patient deal with the illness, cope, and clarify feelings. From Samuel B. Guze, "Psychotherapy and Managed Care," *Archives of General Psychiatry*, Vol. 55 (6), June 1998, pp. 561–62.

167 "The illness is not 'cured'": U.S. Department of Health and Human Services, *Mental Health: A Report of the Surgeon General–Executive Summary*. Rockville, MD: U.S. Department of Health and Human Services, Substance Abuse and Mental Health Services Administration, Center for Mental Health Services, National Institutes of Health, National Institute of Mental Health, 1999.

Chapter 8: Ritalin Nation?

171 Ritalin nation: For this phrase and idea, see Richard DeGrandpre, *Ritalin Nation: Rapid-Fire Culture and the Transformation of Human Consciousness* (New York: W. W. Norton & Co., 1999).

171 "A fourth-grade teacher": Author interview with Wendy Mogel, Author interview, September 13, 2006.

171 "It was patients with high levels of distress": Peter D. Kramer, "Prozac Nation?" *Slate*, February 11, 2008.

172 "The worries expressed about Valium": Author interview with Peter Kramer, Author interview, February 13, 2008.

173 "Anabolic steroids for the soul": Steven Hyman, Quoted in *Beyond Therapy: Biotechnology and the Pursuit of Happiness*, A Report by the President's Council on Bioethics, Washington, D.C., October 15, 2003.

173 "Reclaiming childhood": "Pharmaceutical Companies Find New Ways to Reach Anxious Parents—Go Direct," *San Francisco Chronicle*, December 29, 2003, p. A13.

173 "Back to Basics": Michael Hill, "Parents Make Vintage Nurseries to Take Their Kids Back in Time," Associated Press, April 24, 2006.

174 "Impersonal, competitive . . . self-interested relations": Annette Lareau, *Unequal Childhoods: Class, Race, and Family Life* (Berkeley: University of California Press, 2003), pp. 83 and 247. The phrase "McDonaldization of society" is from the sociologist George Ritzer.

174 "A legitimate concern": Peter N. Stearns, *Anxious Parents: A History of Modern Childrearing in America* (New York: New York University Press, 2003), p. 51.

175 Research now shows parents to be more depressed: Lorraine Ali, "True or False: Having Kids Makes You Happy," newsweek.com, July 7–14, 2008.

177 The average worker's pay: Lynn Brenner, "How Did *You* Do?" Parade.com, March 12, 2006.

177 More than 80 percent of American workers: Ibid.

177 Number of employers offering defined pension plans fell: Families and Work Institute, "2008 National Study of Employers," May 21, 2008.

177 Recent college graduates owed 85 percent more: Lev Grossman, "Grow Up? Not So Fast," *Time*, January 24, 2005, p. 42.

177 Forty percent of students: Carol Smith, "Huge College Loans Eating Up Salaries," seattlepi.com, January 26, 2006 .

178 "Confirm for your child": Sue Shellenbarger, "When Tough Times Weigh on the Kids," wsj.com, September 24, 2008.

178 Stress injuries: Judith Warner, *Perfect Madness: Motherhood in the Age of Anxiety* (New York: Riverhead, 2006), p. 231.

178 Too early specialization: American Academy of Pediatrics, "Intensive Training and Sports Specialization in Young Athletes," *Pediatrics*, Vol. 106 (1), July 2000, pp. 154–57.

178 Sixth-graders: Jody Wilgoren and Jacques Steinberg, "Under Pressure: A Special Report," *The New York Times*, July 3, 2000, p. A1.

178 "Play quotient": Christopher Shea, "Leave Those Kids Alone," boston.com, July 15, 2007.

178 Wealthy parents harass camp directors: Tina Kelley, "Dear Parents—Please Relax, It's Just Camp," *The New York Times*, July 26, 2008.

178 Parents buying spyware: Janet Zimmerman, "Prying Parents," *The Press-Enterprise*, September 4, 2006.

179 Moms and dads edit papers: Barbara Kantrowitz and Peg Tyre, "The Fine Art of Letting Go," newsweek.com, May 14, 2006.

179 Parents accompany recent college graduates: Sue Shellenbarger, "'Kamikaze Parents' at Job Interviews," wsj.com, March 27, 2006.

179 Lori Drew: Judith Warner, "Helicopter Parenting Turns Deadly," nytimes.com, November 11, 2007.

179 Family dinners . . . family vacations have decreased: Alvin Rosenfeld, correspondence with author.

179 Disconnection . . . makes children and teens particularly vulnerable: See, for example, Sharna Olfman, *Childhood Lost: How American Culture Is Failing Our Kids* (Westport, CT: Praeger, 2005), p. 23. Also see the work of Alvin Rosenfeld, Suniya Luthar, Edward M. Hallowell, and many others.

179 Olfman, p. 29.

179 Nearly 40 percent of American workers: National Partnership for Women and Families.

179 Only three states: Christine Vestal, "N.J. Enacts Paid Family Leave," stateline.org, May 14, 2008.

180 Only 16 percent of employers . . . flexibility has declined: The Families and Work Institute, "2008 National Study of Employers," May 21, 2008.

180 Fully three-quarters of Americans: Carolyn B. Maloney, *Rumors of Our Progress Have Been Greatly Exaggerated* (New York: Modern Times, 2008), p. 20.

180 Nearly a third of children: National Association of Child Care Resource and Referral Agencies.

180 Preschool was the single largest expense: Dorie Turner, "Thousands of Families Shut Out of Pre-K Programs," usatoday.com, November 12, 2008.

180 Only eight states plus D.C.: Winnie Hu, "A Promise of Pre-K for All Is Still Far Off in New York," nytimes.com, August 22, 2008.

180 "Sufficiently stimulating experiences": Olfman, p. 28.

180 "Alarmingly unstable": *Perfect Madness*, p. 211.

180 Poor quality day care . . . raises levels of cortisol: See "Excessive Stress Disrupts the Architecture of the Developing Brain," National Scientific Council on the Developing Child, Summer 2005, and Jared A. Lisonbee, "Children's Cortisol and the Quality of Teacher-Child Relationships in Child Care," *Child Development*, Vol. 79 (6), November/December 2008.

181 Almost half of U.S. high school students: Alvin P. Sanoff, "Half of Teens Say School's Unsafe," *USA Today*, August 16, 2005.

181 Kindergarteners are now expected: Peggy Spear, "The Kindergarten Conundrum," *Contra Costa Times*, April 20, 2005.

181 Kindergarteners are required: Richard Rothstein, "Ambitious but Misguided: Kindergarten Academics," *The New York Times*, March 21, 2001, p. B7.

181 Tutors to get kids ready for school: "Cramming for Kindergarten," CBS News, August 12, 2005.

181 "People skills": Ralph Gardner, Jr., "Tot Therapy," *New York*, April 19, 2004, p. 34.

181 Kumon North America: June Kronholz, "Courses Help Kids Get Ready for Kindergarten, Which Is Like First Grade Used to Be," wsj.com, July 12, 2005.

181 In 1981 . . . by 2003: Valerie Strauss, "A Sophisticated Approach," *The Washington Post*, January 18, 2005, p. A6.

181 Lunch was cut: Anand Vaishnav, "School Lunches Are No Picnic," boston.com, August 6, 2005.

181 30,000 elementary schools eliminated recess: David Elkind, *The Power of Play* (Cambridge, MA: Da Capo Press, 2006), p. x.

181 The city of Atlanta: Diane Loupe, "Schools Without Playgrounds," sundaypaper.com, August 5, 2007.

181 71 percent of school districts: Sam Dillon, "Schools Cut Back Subjects to Push Reading and Math," nytimes.com, March 26, 2006.

182 AP courses on Saturdays: Susan Snyder, "Latest Elective: Saturday Classes," philly.com, September 9, 2005.

182 Free time was all but eliminated: In the past twenty years, kids have lost twelve hours per week of free time, eight of which were formerly spent in unstructured play and outdoor activities. David Elkind, *The Power of Play*, Introduction, p. ix.

182 Massive amounts of screen time: Donna St. George, "Getting Lost in the Great Indoors," washingtonpost.com, June 19, 2007.

182 43 percent of babies: Annys Shin, "Diaper Demographic," *The Washington Post*, February 24, 2007, p. D1.

182 "A competitive edge": Carolyn Starks, "More Parents Hiring Personal Trainers for Their Athletic Preteens," *chicagotribune.com*, April 10, 2005.

182 "Enrichment tutoring": Kathleen Carroll, "Costly Tutors on the 'A' list for students," NorthJersey.com, October 23, 2005.

182 "Epidemic of sleep deprivation": Martha Hansen et al., "The Impact of School Daily Schedule on Adolescent Sleep," *Pediatrics*, Vol. 115 (6), June 2005, pp. 1555–561.

182 Children's use of sleeping pills: Gardiner Harris, "Sleeping Pill Use by Youths Soars, Study Says," *The New York Times*, October 19, 2005.

183 Prescription drug *abuse*: "Study: Prescription Abuse Double Since '92," Reuters, CNN.com, July 8, 2005.

183 "Competitive" universities have highest rates of illicit prescription drug use: Donna Leinwand, "Prescription Abusers Not Just After a High," usatoday.com, May 31, 2005.

183 "Not to get high but to feel better": Amy Harmon, "Young, Assured and Playing Pharmacist to Friends," nytimes.com, November 16, 2005.

183 Disconnection: Suniya Luthar, for example, has conducted research linking depression in affluent girls to "isolation from parents." See S. S. Luthar and B. E. Becker, "Privileged But Pressured: A Study of Affluent Youth," *Child Development*, Vol. 73, 2002, pp. 1593–610.

183 "Hyperparenting": According to David Anderegg, professor of psychology at Ben-

nington College, and author of *Worried All the Time: Overparenting in an Age of Anxiety and How to Stop It* (New York: Free Press, 2003).

183 Lenient boundaryless parenting: See, for example, William Damon, director of Stanford University Center on Adolescence, who told *Newsweek*'s Peg Tyre: "The risk of over-indulgence is self-centeredness and self-absorption, and that's a mental-health risk." "The Power of No," *Newsweek*, September 13, 2004, p. 42.

183 Lack of outdoor time: For a full discussion of this, see Richard Louv, *Last Child in the Woods: Saving Our Children from Nature-Deficit Disorder* (Chapel Hill, Algonquin Books of Chapel Hill), 2005.

183 Media use causes lack of imagination: See, for example, Mel Levine, *The Myth of Laziness* (New York: Simon & Schuster, 2003). Also: Excessive television viewing in particular correlates with later attention problems. (Though whether this is a causative relationship or a reflection of the fact that children with attention problems are more likely to watch more TV or to drive their parents to use the TV as a "babysitter" isn't clear. William Stixrud lecture at the Washington Lab School, January 25, 2006.)

183 Early sexualization of girls: American Psychological Association, "Report of the APA Task Force on the Sexualization of Girls," 2007.

183 Too-early academics cause high anxiety and lowered self-esteem: According to Tufts University professor of child development David Elkind in Jodi Helmer, "Tutors for Tots?" *The Christian Science Monitor*, April 5, 2005, p. 14.

183 Yield frustration and anger for preschoolers: Jennifer Steinhauer, "Maybe Preschool Is the Problem," *The New York Times*, May 22, 2005, Section 4, p. 1.

183 Out-of-control kindergarteners: Richard Rothstein, "Ambitious but Misguided: Kindergarten Academics," *The New York Times*, March 21, 2001, p. B7.

184 A lack of development of other human qualities: Dan Kindlon phone interview.

184 Lack of traditional games: Author interview with occupational therapist, Bonnie Eisenson and *New York* magazine: "Marie Leo, an occupational therapist, traces some of her business to children whose coordination is delayed because their preschools are teaching things like computer skills and the position of the planets rather than letting them play."

184 Eating disorders: Nanci Hellmich, "Athletes' hunger to win fuels eating disorders," *USA Today*, February 5, 2006.

184 "Manipulative spin-meisters": Alvin Rosenfeld, "The Over-Scheduled Family," written address provided to author.

184 "One student skipped class": Jonathan D. Glater, "To: Professor@University edu,

Subject: Why It's All About Me," *The New York Times*, February 21, 2006, p. A1.

184 "Pampered, nurtured, and programmed": Stephanie Armour, "Generation Y: They've Arrived at Work with a New Attitude," usatoday.com, November 14, 2005.

185 The Harvard admissions office: William Fitzsimmons, Marlyn McGrath Lewis, and Charles Ducy, "Time Out or Burn Out for the Next Generation," http://www.admissions.college.harvard.edu/apply/time_off/index.html.

185 The *DSM-IV*'s standard: American Psychiatric Association, *Diagnostic and Statistical Manual of Mental Disorders, Fourth Edition*, Washington, D.C., 1994, p. xxi.

185 Stress . . . changes the brain: "Excessive Stress Disrupts the Architecture of the Developing Brain," National Scientific Council on the Developing Child, Summer 2005.

185 "Increasing the risk of stress-related . . . illness": Greg Toppo, "Study: Poverty Dramatically Affects Children's Brains," usatoday.com, December 7, 2008.

185 Chronic stress is believed to lead to depression: Peter Kramer, *Against Depression* (New York:Viking, 2005), p. 118.

186 A "hurried and pressured lifestyle": "For some children, this hurried lifestyle is a source of stress and anxiety and may even contribute to depression," is the AAP position expressed in Kenneth R. Ginsburg, "The Importance of Play in Promoting Healthy Child Development and Maintaining Strong Parent-Child Bonds," *Pediatrics*, Vol. 119 (1), January 2007, pp. 182–91.

186 Fast-track sixth-graders: Jody Wilgoren and Jacques Steinberg, "Under Pressure: A Special Report," *The New York Times*, July 3, 2000, p. A1.

186 Joseph Mahoney: Author interview, October 18, 2006.

186 Twin studies: Brian M. D'Onofrio, Eric Turkheimer et al., "A Children of Twins Study of Parental Divorce and Offspring Psychopathology," *Journal of Child Psychology and Psychiatry*, Vol. 48 (7), 2007, pp. 667–75.

187 Lucky gene variants: Mary Carmichael, "The Resiliency Gene," Newsweek.com, February 5, 2005.

187 New research on intelligence: David L. Kirp, "After the Bell Curve," *The New York Times Magazine*, July 23, 2006, p. 15.

187 Positive caregiving: "Excessive Stress Disrupts the Architecture of the Developing Brain," National Scientific Council on the Developing Child, Summer 2005.

187 "High quality family time": Ginsburg, "The Importance of Play in Promoting

Healthy Child Development and Maintaining Strong Parent-Child Bonds," pp. 182–91.

188 ADT ("attention deficit trait"): Edward M. Hallowell, "Overloaded Circuits: Why Smart People Underperform," *Harvard Business Review*, January 2005, p. 54.

190 "Modern ideas about the innocent child": Gary Cross, *The Cute and the Cool: Wondrous Innocence and Modern American Children's Culture* (New York: Oxford University Press, 2004), p. 206.

Chapter 9: The Stories We Tell

192 Parents who don't believe their kid's disorders are"real": Brea L. Perry, Bernice A. Pescosolido, Jack K. Martin, Jane D. McLeod, and Peter S. Jensen found in "Comparison of Public Attributions, Attitudes, and Stigma in Regard to Depression Among Children and Adults" (*Psychiatric Services*, May 2007, Vol. 58 [5], pp. 632–35), that half the population hadn't heard of ADHD or didn't know much about it; men, blacks, and people with less education knew the least. "However, among those who reported greater knowledge, it was their evaluation of whether ADHD is a 'real' disorder that shaped their endorsement of treatment" (most favored counseling, not meds). Interestingly, they noted, "More respondents saw childhood depression as serious, as needing treatment, and as resulting from underlying genetic or biological problems." Also see Bernice A. Pescosolido, "Culture, Children, and Mental Health Treatment: Special Section on the National Stigma Study-Children," *Psychiatric Services*, Vol. 58 (5), May 2007, pp. 611–12.

193 "Culture of suspicion": Bernice A. Pescosolido, Brea L. Perry, Jack K. Martin, and Jane D. McLeod, "Stigmatizing Attitudes and Beliefs About Treatment and Psychiatric Medications for Children with Mental Illness" *Psychiatric Services*, May 2007, Vol. 58 (5), pp. 613–18.

193 A National Institute of Mental Health report: *Blueprint for Change: Research on Child and Adolescent Mental Health*, Report of the National Advisory Mental Health Council Workgroup on Child and Adolescent Mental Health Intervention Development and Deployment, Washington, D.C.: The National Institute of Mental Health, Office of Communications and Public Liaison, 2001, p. 37.

193 Attitudes have improved modestly: Ramin Mojtabai, "Americans' Attitudes Toward Mental Health Treatment Seeking: 1990–2003," *Psychiatric Services*, Vol. 58 (5), May 2007, pp. 642–51.

193 Forty-five percent . . . 43 percent . . . 35 percent: Pescosolido, Perry, Martin, and McLeod, "Stigmatizing Attitudes and Beliefs About Treatment and Psychiatric Medications for Children with Mental Illness," pp. 613–18.

194 Mental illness and mass murder: In general, said the authors of the National Stigma Study, "the public associates mental illness, particularly depression, with the likelihood of engaging in violent behavior."

194 Eighty-one percent of respondents; 33 percent: Perry, Pescosolido, Martin, McLeod, and Jensen, "Comparison of Public Attributions, Attitudes, and Stigma in Regard to Depression Among Children and Adults," pp. 632–35. Also see Bernice A. Pescosolido, Danielle L. Fettes, Jack K. Martin, John Monahan, Jane D. McLeod, "Perceived Dangerousness of Children with Mental Health Problems and Support for Coerced Treatment," *Psychiatric Services,* Vol. 58, (5), May 2007, pp. 619–25.

194 Indiana University survey: Study was in the *Journal of Health and Social Behavior,* March, 2007. Cited in "Kids with Mental Illness Often Rejected Socially," Reuters, March 19, 2007.

195 "Public perceptions . . . may be more important than evidence": Perry, Pescosolido, Martin, McLeod, and Jensen, "Comparison of Public Attributions, Attitudes, and Stigma in Regard to Depression Among Children and Adults," pp. 632–35.

195 "Popular representations of childhood depression": Ibid.

195 "Legally mandated" treatment: Pescosolido, Fettes, Martin, Monahan, and McLeod, "Perceived Dangerousness of Children with Mental Health Problems and Support for Coerced Treatment," pp. 619–25.

195 More than two-thirds had "negative sentiments": Pescosolido, Perry, Martin, and McLeod, "Stigmatizing Attitudes and Beliefs About Treatment and Psychiatric Medications for Children with Mental Illness," pp. 613–18.

195 "Concern for parental responsibility": Pescosolido, Fettes, Martin, Monahan, and McLeod, "Perceived Dangerousness of Children with Mental Health Problems and Support for Coerced Treatment," pp. 619–25.

196 Because of stigma, many don't seek services: "Services cannot be effective for families concerned about stigma because these families are unlikely to access available resources or accept recommended treatment options," write Pescosolido, Perry, Martin, and McLeod, "Stigmatizing Attitudes and Beliefs About Treatment and Psychiatric Medications for Children with Mental Illness," pp. 613–18.

196 "A scourge": Ken Kusmer, "Six Counties to Screen Youth Offenders for Mental Illness," Associated Press State & Local Wire, June 7, 2007.

198 "A bottomless pit": Bob Berger, "A Journey Toward Hope," parenting.com.

201 "Devastating effects": Perry, Pescosolido, Martin, McLeod, and Jensen, "Comparison of Public Attributions, Attitudes, and Stigma in Regard to Depression Among Children and Adults," pp. 632–35.

201 William Bruce: Elizabeth Bernstein and Nathan Koppel, "A Death in the Family," *The Wall Street Journal*, August 16, 2008.

203 ADHD . . . no lasting effect: See, for example, Benedict Carey, "Bad Behavior Does Not Doom Pupils, Studies Say," *The New York Times*, November 13, 2007.

204 "It's bad for the brain to be mentally ill": Author interview with John March, February 20, 2009.

204 Fully two-thirds of children with ADHD: Author interview with Philip Shaw, November 14, 2007.

204 Untreated children with ADHD: "International Consensus Statement on ADHD," *Clinical Child and Family Psychology Review*, Vol. 5 (2), June 2002, pp. 89–111.

205 "Mismanage or endanger their lives": Ibid.

205 If they receive proper treatment: Pamela White, "Autism Epidemic," *Boulder Weekly*, April 12, 2007.

205 Depression is toxic for the developing brain: Peter Kramer, *Against Depression* (New York: Viking, 2005), p. 118.

205 "It scars the brain": Author interview with William Stixrud, September 26, 2006.

206 "Parents don't make their children sick": Harold S. Koplewicz, *It's Nobody's Fault: New Hope and Help for Difficult Children and Their Parents* (New York: Times Books, 1996), p. xii.

Chapter 10: A "Better Time Than Ever"

209 "Just thirty years ago": Roy Richard Grinker, *Unstrange Minds: Remapping the World of Autism* (Cambridge: Basic Books, 2007), p. 5–6.

210 "Medicines": Stories on this abound. See, for example, Jane Gross, "Checklist for Camp: Bug Spray. Sunscreen. Pills," *The New York Times*, July 16, 2006.

211 Antidepressants, coupled with cognitive behavioral therapy, work: Author interview with John March, February 20, 2009.

211 Studies that show antidepressants don't work: See, for example, Irving Kirsch et al., "Initial Severity and Antidepressant Benefits: A Meta-Analysis of

Data Submitted to the Food and Drug Administration," *PLoS Med*, Vol. 5 (2), February 26, 2008.

211 Stimulant medications are effective for 70 to 80 percent of kids: NYU Child Study Center, "Facts About Children and Adolescents with ADHD," aboutourkids org.

212 "A major public health success story": Darshak Sanghavi, "Ritalin Fears Overblown," *The Boston Globe*, April 26, 2005, p. E1.

212 "Children with obsessive-compulsive disorder": John March, "The Future of Psychotherapy for Mentally Ill Children and Adolescents," *The Journal of Child Psychology and Psychiatry*, Vol. 50 (1–2), 2009.

212 Children with dyslexia: "Recent advances in dyslexia provide a developmentally sound framework for understanding how the treatment of disordered phonological processing with a psychosocial intervention (intensive tutoring) works directly on the brain by elaborating compensatory neurocircuitry." John S. March, "The Future of Psychotherapy for Mentally Ill Children and Adolescents," pp. 170–79.

212 One 2007 report: Steven Carter and Amy Hsuan, "Record Number in Special Ed," *The Oregonian*, February 15, 2007.

212 "From the era of blame and shame": Author interview with Thomas Insel, Author interview, February 24, 2009.

214 The work of developmental neuroscience: Psychosocial interventions "aim to restore normal developmental process or to initiate compensatory processes that return a patient to a functional neurodevelopmental trajectory," writes John March in "The Future of Psychotherapy for Mentally Ill Children and Adolescents," pp. 170–79.

215 The results are very mixed: Michael T. Compton, "Advances in Early Intervention in the Prodromal Phase of Schizophrenia," Coverage of American Psychiatric Association 2005 Meeting, medscape.com. And Tonya White, Afshan Anjum, and S. Charles Schultz, "The Schizophrenia Prodrome," *American Journal of Psychiatry*, Vol. 163, March 2006, pp. 376–80.

215 What differentiates the brains of kids with bipolar disorder: Ellen Leibenluft, "Pediatric Bipolar Disorder Comes of Age," *Archives of General Psychiatry*, Vol. 65 (10), 2008, pp. 1122–24, and interviews with Ellen Leibenluft, September 24, 2008 and March 3, 2009.

216 Fragile X: Interview with John March. Also see, for example, Jon Hamilton, "Drugs Hint at Potential Reversal of Autism," npr.org, October 15, 2008.

217 Stimulant medications *may* restore: Interview with Thomas Insel, director of the National Institute of Mental Health, February 24, 2009. Also: "If you take stimulants, your central nervous system looks more normal than if you don't, and the brain develops more normally if you have stimulants," March said.

217 Drugs that could specifically help shield: Peter Kramer, *Against Depression* (New York: Viking, 2005), p. 191 ff.

219 Only a third of the treatments: Benedict Carey, "Most Will Be Mentally Ill at Some Point, Study Says," *The New York Times*, June 7, 2005, p. A17.

219 Eight to twelve minutes: According to a 2003 survey conducted by Children's National Medical Center, cited in "National Survey of Pediatricians Says Time Restraints Affect Quality of Medical Care for Children," U.S. Newswire, February 4, 2003.

219 The most extensive study on ADHD treatment: The MTA Cooperative Group, "A 14-month randomized clinical trial of treatment strategies for attention-deficit/hyperactivity disorder," *Archives of General Psychiatry*, Vol. 56, 1999, pp. 1073–86.

220 And 2007: The MTA Cooperative Group, "National Institute of Mental Health Multimodal Treatment Study of ADHD Follow-up: Changes in Effectiveness and Growth After the End of Treatment," *Pediatrics*, Vol. 113 (4), April 2004, pp. 762–69.

220 Their behavior actually became "normal": Peter S. Jensen et al., "3-Year Follow-up of the NIMH MTA Study," *Journal of the American Academy of Child & Adolescent Psychiatry*, Vol. 46 (8), August 2007, pp. 988–1000.
Interview with Peter Jensen, October 22, 2008.

220 Only a "small proportion" of doctors: William Frankenberger, Carey Farmer, Laura Parker, and Joe Cermak, "The Use of Stimulant Medication for Treatment of Attention-Deficit/Hyperactivity Disorder: A survey of school psychologists' knowledge, attitudes, and experience," Developmental Disabilities Bulletin, 2001, Vol. 29 (2), pp. 132–51.

221 Parents were most satisfied: The MTA Cooperative Group, "National Institute of Mental Health Multimodal Treatment Study of ADHD Follow-up: Changes in Effectiveness and Growth After the End of Treatment," pp. 762–69.

221 Learned to get along better with their parents: Jensen interview. Parent/child interactions is the one area where therapy does better than medication.

221 Kids just get medication: One 2008 study that tracked the care of 6.8 million children and teens from 2002 to 2006 found that almost 60 percent of the kids who were treated for depression received antidepressants with no therapy at all,

despite repeated studies having found that teens who get cognitive behavioral therapy along with medication reap much greater benefits, with lesser risks. Marilyn Elias, "Study: Most Depressed Kids Get Antidepressants but No Therapy," *USA Today*, October 8, 2008. Another study that year found that, despite all the publicity surrounding antidepressants and suicide, only 3 percent of teenagers diagnosed with depression and prescribed medication were getting the number of follow-up visits considered necessary to monitor them for side effects like increased suicidal thoughts. Josephine Marcotty, "Depressed Teens on Meds Lack Scrutiny," StarTribune.com, February 6, 2008.

221 Kids end up on multiple medications: One 2005 study showed 40 percent of child psychiatric patients taking two or more medications. Farifteh Firoozmand Duffy et al., "Concomitant Pharmacotherapy Among Youths Treated in Routine Psychiatric Practice," *Journal of Child and Adolescent Psychopharmacology*, Vol. 15 (1), 2005, pp. 12–25.

221 There's no solid evidence: According to John S. March et al., "The Case for Practical Clinical Trials in Psychiatry," *American Journal of Psychiatry*, Vol. 162, 2005, pp. 836–46, the scientific support for the use of multiple medications in children is "completely lacking."

222 Fractured the delivery of mental health care: Samuel B. Guze, "Psychotherapy and Managed Care," *Archives of General Psychiatry*, Vol. 55 (6), June 1998, pp. 561–62.

223 "Ineffective, controversial methods of treatment": American Academy of Pediatrics, "Joint Statement—Learning Disabilities, Dyslexia, and Vision," *Pediatrics*, Vol. 124 (2), August 2009, p. 842.

224 "We needed help from someone": Paul Raeburn, *Acquainted with the Night* (New York: Broadway Books, 2005), pp. 7–8.

231 "Love and support": Author interview with Peter Jensen, October 22, 2008.

Chapter 11: Moving Forward

236 A "pattern of recurrent moral panics": Steven Mintz, *Huck's Raft: A History of American Childhood* (Cambridge: Belknap Press, 2004), p. ix.

236 A "misplaced sense of crisis": Ibid., p. 336.

236 "Children have long served": Ibid., p. 340.

237 An insidious level of hostility: Ginia Bellafante, "Children, Apples of Parents' Eyes, Face Arrows on TV," *The New York Times*, November 19, 2005.

237 "The literature of children in peril": Ginia Bellafante, "Jodi Picoult and the Anxious Parent," *The New York Times*, June 17, 2009.

239 A "religious war": Shorter cited in Benedict Carey, "Panel to Weigh Expansion of Antidepressant Warnings," *The New York Times*, December 13, 2006, p. A26.

239 A "medical home": Phrase is from pediatrician John Stirling and child psychiatrist Lisa Amaya-Jackson, "Understanding the Behavioral and Emotional Consequences of Child Abuse," *Pediatrics*, Vol. 122, (3), September 2008.

241 They slip through the cracks: Lidia Wasowicz, "Ped Med: Young Minds Under Attack," United Press International, January 9, 2006.

242 Clean up their acts: Duff Wilson, "Harvard Medical School in Ethics Quandary," *The New York Times*, March 3, 2009.

242 The NYU Child Study Center: Author interview with Harold Koplewicz, head of NYU Child Study Center.

242 The University of Pittsburgh School of Medicine: Gardiner Harris, "Ban Urged on Gifts at Medical Schools," *The New York Times*, April 28, 2008.

242 Mayo Clinic: Gardiner Harris, Benedict Carey, and Janet Roberts, "Psychiatrists, Children, and Drug Industry's Role," *The New York Times*, May 10, 2007.

242 Nearly four times as likely: Marcia Angell, *The Truth About the Drug Companies* (New York: Random House, 2004), p. 106.

243 90 percent cure rate: According to Dr. Xavier Castellanos (Professor of Child and Adolescent Psychiatry; Director of Research; Director, Phyllis Green and Randolph Ćowen Institute for Pediatric Neuroscience; Professor of Radiology New York University Medical School) interviewed on *Frontline*, "The Medicated Child," January 8, 2008.

244 Congress has begun: "Countering the Drug Salesmen," (editorial) *The New York Times*, March 20, 2008.

244 Some legislators: Natasha Singer, "Lawmakers Seek to Curb Drug Commercials," *The New York Times*, July 27, 2009.

245 "Disclosure may be used to 'sanitize'": A. Brennan Troyen et al., "Health Industry Practices That Create Conflicts of Interest," *JAMA*, Vol. 295, 2006, pp. 429–33.

246 Spending . . . nearly tripled: Angell, p. 123.

246 Pressures on physicians: Cindy Parks Thomas et al., "Trends in the Use of Psychotropic Medications Among Adolescents, 1994 to 2001," *Psychiatric Services*, Vol. 57 (1), January 2006, pp. 63–69.

247 The horrifically punitive way: Ashley Fantz, "Children Forced into Cell-like Seclusion Rooms," CNN.com, January 8, 2009.

Bibliography

American Psychiatric Association. *Diagnostic and Statistical Manual: Mental Disorders.* 1952.

——. *Diagnostic and Statistical Manual of Mental Disorders, Second Edition.* 1968.

Angell, Marcia. *The Truth About the Drug Companies.* New York: Random House, 2004.

Barber, Charles. *Comfortably Numb: How Psychiatry Is Medicating a Nation.* New York: Pantheon Books, 2008.

Barkley, Russell A. *Taking Charge of ADHD: The Complete, Authoritative Guide for Parents.* New York: Guilford Press, 1995.

Berlin, Richard M., ed. *Poets on Prozac: Mental Illness, Treatment and the Creative Process.* Baltimore: Johns Hopkins University Press, 2008.

Beyond Therapy: Biotechnology and the Pursuit of Happiness. A report by the President's Council on Bioethics, Washington, D.C., October 15, 2003.

Blueprint for Change: Research on Child and Adolescent Mental Health. Report of the National Advisory Mental Health Council Workgroup on Child and Adolescent Mental Health Intervention Development and Deployment. Washington, D.C.: The National Institute of Mental Health, Office of Communications and Public Liaison, 2001.

Breggin, Peter R., and Ginger Ross Breggin. *The War Against Children.* New York: St. Martin's, 1994.

Brodey, Denise, ed. *The Elephant in the Playroom: Ordinary Parents Write Intimately and Honestly About the Extraordinary Highs and Heartbreaking Lows of Raising Kids with Special Needs.* New York: Hudson Street Press, 2007.

Cerullo, Michael A. "Cosmetic Psychopharmacology and the President's Council on Bioethics." *Perspectives in Biology and Medicine,* Volume 49 (4), Autumn 2006, pp. 515–23.

Conrad, Peter. *The Medicalization of Society: On the Transformation of Human Conditions into Treatable Disorders*. Baltimore: Johns Hopkins University Press, 2007.

Cross, Gary. *The Cute and the Cool: Wondrous Innocence and Modern American Children's Culture*. New York: Oxford University Press, 2004.

DeGrandpre, Richard. *The Cult of Pharmacology: How America Became the World's Most Troubled Drug Culture*. Durham: Duke University Press, 2006.

——. *Ritalin Nation: Rapid-Fire Culture and the Transformation of Human Consciousness*. New York: W. W. Norton & Co., 1999.

"Diagnosis and Treatment of Attention Deficit Hyperactivity Disorder." National Institutes of Health Consensus Development Conference Statement. November 16–18, 1998, http://consensus.nih.gov/1998/1998AttentionDeficitHyperactivityDisorder110html.htm

Diala, Chamberlain, Carles Muntaner, Christine Walrath, Kim J. Nickerson, Thomas A. LaVeist, and Philip J. Leaf. "Racial Differences in Attitudes Toward Professional Mental Health Care and in the Use of Services." *American Journal of Orthopsychiatry*. Vol. 70 (4), October 2000, pp. 455–464.

Diller, Lawrence H. *The Last Normal Child: Essays on the Intersection of Kids, Culture and Psychiatric Drugs*. Westport, CT: Praeger, 2006.

——. *Should I Medicate My Child?* New York: Basic Books, 2002.

Eberstadt, Mary. *Home-Alone America: The Hidden Toll of Day Care, Behavioral Drugs, and Other Parent Substitutes*. New York: Sentinel, 2004.

Elliott, Carl. *Better Than Well: American Medicine Meets the American Dream*. New York: W. W. Norton & Co., 2003.

Faber, Adele, and Elaine Mazlish. *Liberated Parents, Liberated Children*. New York: Grosset and Dunlap, 1974.

Ford, Anne. *Laughing Allegra*. New York: Newmarket Press, 2003.

Fraiberg, Selma H. *The Magic Years*. New York: Scribner's, 1959.

Garbarino, James. *Lost Boys: Why Our Sons Turn Violent and How We Can Save Them*. New York: Free Press, 1999.

Geller, Barbara, Bitsy Zimmerman, Merlene Williams, Melissa P. DelBello, Jeanne Fraxier, and Linda Beringer. "Phenomenology of Prepubertal and Early Adolescent Bipolar Disorder: Examples of Elated Mood, Grandiose Behaviors, Decreased Need for Sleep, Racing Thoughts and Hypersexuality." *Journal of Child and Adolescent Psychopharmacology*. Vol. 12 (1), 2002, pp. 3–9.

Gleick, James. *Faster: The Acceleration of Just About Everything*. New York: Pantheon, 1999.

Glenmullen, Joseph. *Prozac Backlash: Overcoming the Angers of Prozac, Zoloft, Paxil and other Antidepressants with Safe, Effective Alternatives.* New York: Simon & Schuster, 2000.

Golden, Daniel. *The Price of Admission: How America's Ruling Class Buys Its Way Into Elite Colleges–And Who Gets Left Outside the Gates.* New York: Crown, 2006.

Greenberg, Joanne. *I Never Promised You a Rose Garden.* New York: Signet, 1964.

Greenberg, Rosalie. *Bipolar Kids: Helping Your Child Find Calm in the Mood Storm.* Cambridge, MA: Da Capo Press, 2007.

Greenspan, Stanley. *The Secure Child: Helping Children Feel Safe and Confident in a Changing World.* Cambridge, MA: Da Capo Press, 2002.

Grinker, Roy Richard. *Unstrange Minds: Remapping the World of Autism.* Cambridge, MA: Basic Books, 2007.

Guevara, James P., Chris Feudtner, Daniel Romer, Thomas Power, Ricardo Eiraldi, Snejana Nitianova, Aracely Rosales, Janet Ohene-Frempong, and Donald F. Schwarz, "Fragmented Care for Inner-City Minority Children with Attention-Deficit/Hyperactivity Disorder." *Pediatrics.* Vol. 116 (4), October 2005, pp. 512–17.

Hallowell, Edward M. *The Childhood Roots of Adult Happiness.* New York: Ballantine Books, 2002.

——. *CrazyBusy: Overstretched, Overbooked, and About to Snap!* New York: Ballantine Books, 2006.

Hartmann, Thom. *Beyond ADD: Hunting for Reasons in the Past and Present.* Grass Valley, CA: Underwood Books, 1996.

Hawes, Joseph, and N. Ray Himer, eds. *American Childhood: A Research Guide and Historical Handbook.* Westport, CT: Greenwood Press, 1985.

Healy, David. *The Antidepressant Era.* Cambridge, MA: Harvard University Press, 1997.

——. *The Creation of Psychopharmacology.* Cambridge, MA: Harvard University Press, 2002.

——. *Let Them Eat Prozac: The Unhealthy Relationship Between the Pharmaceutical Industry and Depression.* New York: New York University Press, 2004.

Horwitz, Allan V. *Creating Mental Illness.* Chicago: University of Chicago Press, 2002.

Horwitz, Allan V., and Jerome C. Wakefield. *The Loss of Sadness: How Psychiatry Transformed Normal Sorrow into Depressive Disorder.* New York: Oxford University Press, 2007.

Howe, Neil, and William Strauss. *Millennials Rising: The Next Great Generation.* New York: Vintage, 2000.

Huxley, Aldous. *The Doors of Perception and Heaven and Hell.* New York: Harper Colophon, 1963.

Kesey, Ken. *One Flew Over the Cuckoo's Nest.* New York: Penguin, 2002.

Kindlon, Dan. *Too Much of a Good Thing: Raising Children of Character in an Indulgent Age.* New York: Hyperion, 2001.

Klass, Perri, and Eileen Costello. *Quirky Kids: Understanding and Helping Your Child Who Doesn't Fit In—When to Worry and When* Not *to Worry.* New York: Ballantine Books, 2003.

Koplewicz, Harold S. *It's Nobody's Fault: New Hope and Help for Difficult Children and Their Parents.* New York: Times Books, 1996.

Kos, Julie M., Amanda L. Richdale, and David A. Hay. "Children with Attention Deficit Hyperactivity Disorder and Their Teachers: A Review of the Literature." *International Journal of Disability, Development and Education.* Vol. 53 (2), June 2006, pp. 147–60.

Kramer, Peter D. *Against Depression.* New York: Viking, 2005.

——. *Listening to Prozac: A Psychiatrist Explores Antidepressant Drugs and the Remaking of the Self.* New York: Viking, 1993.

Kranowitz, Carol Stock. *The Out-of-Sync Child: Recognizing and Coping with Sensory Integration Dysfunction.* New York: Perigee, 1998.

Kutchins, Herb, and Stuart A. Kirk. *Making Us Crazy: DSM: The Psychiatric Bible and the Creation of Mental Disorders.* New York: The Free Press, 1997.

Lane, Christopher. *Shyness: How Normal Behavior Became a Sickness.* New Haven: Yale University Press, 2007.

Lareau, Annette. *Unequal Childhoods: Class, Race and Family Life.* Berkeley, CA: University of California Press, 2003.

LeFever, Gretchen B., Keila V. Dawson, and Ardythe L. Morrow. "The Extent of Drug Therapy for Attention Deficit-Hyperactivity Disorder Among Children in Public Schools." *American Journal of Public Health.* Vol. 89 (9), September 1999, pp. 1359–364.

Leibenluft, Ellen. "Pediatric Bipolar Disorder Comes of Age." *Archives of General Psychiatry.* Vol. 65 (10), 2008, pp. 1122–24.

Kalikow, Kevin T. *Your Child in the Balance: An Insider's Guide for Parents to the Psychiatric Medication Dilemma.* New York: Perseus, 2006.

Kessler, Jane W. *Psychopathology of Childhood.* Second Edition. Englewood Cliffs, NJ: Prentice Hall, 1988.

Leslie, Laurel K., Jill Weckerly, John Landsverk, Richard L. Hough, Michael S. Hurlburt, and Patricia A. Wood. "Racial/Ethnic Differences in the Use of Psychotropic Medication in High-Risk Children and Adolescents." *Journal of the American Academy of Child & Adolescent Psychiatry.* Vol. 42 (23), December 2003, pp. 1433–42.

Levine, Madeline. *The Price of Privilege: How Parental Pressure and Material Advantage Are Creating a Generation of Disconnected and Unhappy Kids.* New York: HarperCollins, 2006.

Levine, Mel. *A Mind at a Time.* New York: Simon & Schuster, 2002.

——. *The Myth of Laziness.* New York: Simon & Schuster, 2003.

Marano, Hara Estroff. *A Nation of Wimps: The High Cost of Invasive Parenting.* New York: Broadway Books, 2008.

Mental Health: A Report of the Surgeon General. Washington, D.C.: Department of Health and Human Services, 1999. See, in particular, Chapter 3, "Children and Mental Health."

Metzl, Jonathan Michel. *Prozac on the Couch: Prescribing Gender in the Era of Wonder Drugs.* Durham and London: Duke University Press, 2003.

Mintz, Steven. *Huck's Raft: A History of American Childhood.* Cambridge, MA: Belknap Press, 2004.

Moynihan, Ray, and Alan Cassels. *Selling Sickness: How the World's Biggest Pharmaceutical Companies Are Turning Us All Into Patients.* New York: Nation Books, 2005.

MTA Cooperative Group. "National Institute of Mental Health Multimodal Treatment Study of ADHD Follow-up: Changes in Effectiveness and Growth After the End of Treatment." *Pediatrics,* Vol. 113 (4), April 2004, pp. 762–69.

——. "National Institute of Mental Health Multimodal Treatment Study of ADHD Follow-up: 24-Month Outcomes of Treatment Strategies for Attention-Deficit/Hyperactivity Disorder." *Pediatrics,* Vol. 113 (4), April 2004, pp. 754–61.

Olfman, Sharna, ed. *Childhood Lost: How American Culture Is Failing Our Kids.* Westport, CT: Praeger, 2005.

Olfson, Mark, Marc J. Gameroff, Steven C. Marcus, and Peter S. Jensen. "National Trends in the Treatment of Attention Deficit Hyperactivity Disorder." *The American Journal of Psychiatry.* Vol. 160 (6), June 2003, pp. 1071–77.

Papolos, Demitri and Janice. *The Bipolar Child.* New York: Broadway Books, 2002.

Pelham, William E., et al. "Behavioral versus Behavioral and Pharmacological Treatment in ADHD Children Attending a Summer Treatment Program." *Journal of Abnormal Child Psychology.* Vol. 28 (6), 2000, pp. 507–25.

Postman, Neil. *The Disappearance of Childhood.* New York: Delacorte, 1982.

Raeburn, Paul. *Acquainted with the Night: A Parent's Quest to Understand Depression and Bipolar Disorder in His Children.* New York: Broadway Books, 2005.

Report of the Working Group on Psychotropic Medications for Children and Adolescents. American Psychological Association, 2006.

Rosemond, John, and Bose Ravenel. *The Diseasing of America's Children.* Nashville, TN: Thomas Nelson, 2008.

Rutter, Michael, Eric Taylor, and Lionel Sersov, eds. *Child and Adolescent Psychiatry: Modern Approaches.* Oxford: Blackwell Sciences, 1994.

Schnittker, Jason. "Misgivings of Medicine? African Americans' Skepticism of Psychiatric Medication." *Journal of Health and Social Behavior.* Vol. 44, December 2003, pp. 506–24.

Schnittker, Jason, Jeremy Freese, and Brian Powell. "Nature, Nurture, Neither, Nor: Black-White Differences in Beliefs About the Causes and Appropriate Treatment of Mental Illness." *Social Forces.* Vol. 78 (3), March 2000, pp. 1101–130.

Schor, Juliet. *Born to Buy: The Commercialized Child and the New Consumer Culture.* New York: Scribner, 2004.

Sealander, Judith. *The Failed Century of the Child: Governing America's Young in the Twentieth Century.* Cambridge, MA: Cambridge University Press, 2003.

Shorter, Edward. *A History of Psychiatry: From the Era of the Asylum to the Age of Prozac.* New York: John Wiley & Sons, 1997.

Spencer, Thomas J., Joseph Biederman, Janet Wozniak, Stephen V. Faraone, Timothy E. Wilens, and Eric Mick. "Parsing Pediatric Bipolar Disorder from Its Associated Comorbidity with the Disruptive Behavior Disorders." *Biological Psychiatry.* Vol. 49, 2001, pp. 1062–70.

Spiegel, Alix. "The Dictionary of Disorder: How One Man Revolutionized Psychiatry." *The New Yorker.* January 3, 2005.

Spock, Benjamin. *A Better World for Our Children.* Bethesda, MD: National Press Books, 1994.

Stearns, Peter N. *Anxious Parents: A History of Modern Childrearing in America.* New York: New York University Press, 2003.

Stevens, Jack, Jeffrey S. Harman, and Kelly J. Kelleher. "Race/Ethnicity and Insurance Status as Factors Associated with ADHD Treatment Patterns." *Journal of Child and Adolescent Psychopharmacology.* Vol. 15 (1), 2005, pp. 88–96.

Szasz, Thomas. *The Medicalization of Everyday Life: Selected Essays.* Syracuse, NY: Syracuse University Press, 2007.

——. *Psychiatry: The Science of Lies.* Syracuse, NY: Syracuse, University Press, 2008.

Thompson, Vetta L. Sanders, Anita Bazile, and Maysa Akbar. "African Americans' Perceptions of Psychotherapy and Psychotherapists." *Professional Psychology: Research and Practice.* Vol. 35 (10), pp. 19–26.

Tone, Andrea. *The Age of Anxiety: A History of America's Turbulent Affair with Tranquilizers.* New York: Basic Books, 2008.

Twenge, Jean. *Generation Me: Why Today's Young Americans Are More Confident, Assertive, Entitled–and More Miserable Than Ever Before.* New York: Free Press, 2006.

Wilson, Eric G. *Against Happiness.* New York: Farrar, Straus & Giroux, 2008.

Index